T0301127

ĀYURVEDA IN YOGA TEACHING

Yoga Teaching Guides

As it grows in popularity, teaching yoga requires an increasing set of skills and understanding, in terms of both yoga practice and knowledge. This series of books guides you towards becoming an accomplished, trusted yoga teacher by refining your teaching skills and methods. The series, written by experts in the field, focuses on the key topics for yoga teachers – including sequencing, language in class, anatomy and running a successful and thriving yoga business – and presents practical information in an accessible manner and format for all levels. Each book is filled with visual aids to enhance the reading experience, and includes 'top tips' to highlight and emphasize key ideas and advice.

in the same series

Supporting Yoga Students with Common Injuries and Conditions
A Handbook for Teachers and Trainees
Dr. Andrew McGonigle
ISBN 978 1 78775 469 0
eISBN 978 1 78775 470 6

Qigong in Yoga Teaching and Practice
Understanding Qi and the Use of Meridian Energy
Joo Teoh
Foreword by Mimi Kuo-Deemer
ISBN 978 1 78775 652 6
eISBN 978 1 78775 653 3

Developing a Yoga Home Practice
An Exploration for Yoga Teachers and Trainees
Alison Leighton with Joe Taft
ISBN 978 1 78775 704 2
eISBN 978 1 78775 705 9

Theming Skills for Yoga Teachers
Tools to Inspire Creative and Connected Classes
Tanja Mickwitz
ISBN 978 1 78775 687 8
eISBN 978 1 78775 688 5

of related interest

Yoga Teaching Handbook
A Practical Guide for Yoga Teachers and Trainees
Edited by Sian O'Neill
ISBN 978 1 84819 355 0
eISBN 978 0 85701 313 2

Yoga Student Handbook
Develop Your Knowledge of Yoga Principles and Practice
Edited by Sian O'Neill
Foreword by Lizzie Lasater
ISBN 978 0 85701 386 6
eISBN 978 0 85701 388 0

ĀYURVEDA IN YOGA TEACHING

Tarik Dervish

Illustrations by Masha Pimas

Series Editor: Sian O'Neill

SINGING DRAGON
LONDON AND PHILADELPHIA

First published in Great Britain in 2022 by Singing Dragon,
an imprint of Jessica Kingsley Publishers
An Hachette Company

2

Copyright © Tarik Dervish 2022

The right of Tarik Dervish to be identified as the Author of the Work has been asserted by him in accordance with the Copyright, Designs and Patents Act 1988.

Illustrations copyright © Masha Pimas 2022

All rights reserved. No part of this publication may be reproduced, stored in a retrieval system, or transmitted, in any form or by any means without the prior written permission of the publisher, nor be otherwise circulated in any form of binding or cover other than that in which it is published and without a similar condition being imposed on the subsequent purchaser.

All pages marked with can be photocopied and downloaded for personal use with this programme, but may not be reproduced for any other purposes without the permission of the publisher.

The information contained in this book is not intended to replace the services of trained medical professionals or to be a substitute for medical advice. The complementary therapy described in this book may not be suitable for everyone to follow. You are advised to consult a doctor before embarking on any complementary therapy programme and on any matters relating to your health, and in particular on any matters that may require diagnosis or medical attention.

A CIP catalogue record for this title is available from the British Library and the Library of Congress

ISBN 978 1 78775 595 6
eISBN 978 1 78775 596 3

Printed and bound in Great Britain by Clays Ltd

Jessica Kingsley Publishers' policy is to use papers that are natural, renewable and recyclable products and made from wood grown in sustainable forests. The logging and manufacturing processes are expected to conform to the environmental regulations of the country of origin.

Jessica Kingsley Publishers
Carmelite House
50 Victoria Embankment
London EC4Y 0DZ

www.singingdragon.com

CONTENTS

ACKNOWLEDGEMENTS

I would like to acknowledge the generations of seers and teachers who tirelessly passed the light of this amazing knowledge down through the generations of the many seekers and precious finders. Without their dedicated efforts, our suffering would have been much greater. Now, I feel the weight of this responsibility to ensure that future generations of students are guided properly to ensure that the knowledge remains as relevant now as it was thousands of years ago.

A special thanks to all the wonderful teachers who have helped me navigate the ever-evolving map of wisdom and insight into the nature of reality. The map seems to change with every new insight, but when I look more closely, the map actually remains the same. It is my eyes and mind that do not see what has always been there.

I thank my father (RIP) who was my first spiritual teacher, and as I age and encounter new teachers, his wisdom echoes again and again in different voices.

I would like to thank Dr David Frawley. His books and teachings have given me great clarity on the Vedic perspective of Āyurveda for many decades.

A huge thank you to Dr Vasant Lad, the great luminary with whom I was blessed to study every year for over ten years at the Bhaktivedanta Manor in Watford. His teachings have helped me enormously in understanding the huge scope and application of Āyurveda, particularly for western students.

I thank all the teachers who bravely introduced Āyurveda to the UK as a serious study at university level. Without them, I would not have had the opportunity to learn about it at such depth.

A special thank you to Pavlos Mastihi (RIP) for supporting my work and my life and being a great friend. He took the photo used for the cover of this book and many others. Unfortunately, his soul didn't hang around long enough to see the publication of this book. May he rest in peace.

I thank all my family, friends and colleagues who have made the journey less lonely and helped to keep the flame of Āyurveda alive over the years. Āyurveda has grown both in stature and importance and there are more opportunities to benefit from it now than ever before.

A big thank you to Masha Pimas for creating such great illustrations for this book.

Finally, a big thank you to my editor, Sian O'Neill, who supported the writing and publication of this book. She believed in my vision and recognized a need for what this book will share.

PREFACE

My yoga journey

My life has been easy except that someone forgot to tell me. They forgot to tell me that given half the chance, I would have grown to like and honour myself, my natural inclinations would have been celebrated and I would have glided through life without any crippling health problems.

I suffered from many emotional problems as a teen and into my 20s and caused myself a great deal of physical upset by over-exercising and hurting my back at the tender age of 18. We think we are invincible at that age until something goes horribly wrong and we end up paying for it for the rest of our lives. That was me, unfortunately. I sort of blame myself in the shoulda-woulda-coulda sort of way, but I was young, not well guided, very emotionally unsupported (this was the 1980s, after all) and, well, the rest is a missed-story. Missed opportunities to grow and shine in the way a bright young person should.

But looking back, I can see that I grew strong in other ways. I developed a sensitivity and empathy that was uncommon in someone so young and this helped shaped my identity.

I came into meditation before yoga. When I was 17, my late father introduced me to a spiritual organization called the Divine Light Movement, today known as The Prem Rawat Foundation. I wouldn't say it changed my life exactly but what I do recognize is that I was given an extremely powerful tool for coping with life's ups and downs. Because I had a regular meditation practice and a supportive community of *premis* (as they were then called) I didn't get quite as drunk as my peers and managed to avoid many scrapes. I used to practise every damned day and it put me in a mental space that slowly changed my perception of reality completely.

I think all young people live in a state of semi-magical realism because that's part of what being young is all about. You create a version of life in your head that is full of romance and possibility. Everything is new and exciting, and everyone is a kind of extension of your imagined self. I was lucky enough to be immersed in big ideas at that time too. My first degree was in Modern Languages and Literature. French existentialism and Spanish pantheism infused my sense of reality with a deep sense of wonder. The most magical thing about being a not-yet-formed person is that your connection with the mind and senses is also in a malleable state. You are still negotiating your reality. The conditions of the material world, of having to earn a living and all the rest, eventually force any fanciful edifices to come crashing down for most of us and as the years roll on, we salvage what we can from the wreckage.

I labelled myself a 'seeker' when I looked back at my choices and realized that at regular junctions in my life, I felt compelled to *seek*. Seeking what? Well, happiness in short. I was convinced that my dis-ease was a puzzle to be solved. What I was yearning for was the secret to a fulfilled life. The secret to feeling whole. That's why science never attracted me. I was never inspired by the idea of knowing why what went up had to come down, or why aeroplanes could stay in the air for so long. I somehow didn't care. I believed that the missing jigsaw pieces could be found in traditional fields of knowledge, so that's where my attention went.

If meditation could do that much for me, what other marvels awaited me? I immersed myself in the study of western astrology, which blew my mind for many years, until I found myself where I started, which was not quite satisfied, incomplete. At the same time, I threw myself into all things yoga. I discovered āsana, prāṇāyāma, mudrā, bandha, mantra, yantra… what an adventure! I felt like I was being fed the food of the gods.

But I was still unwell, and it was getting me down. I had digestive problems, recurring back pain and depression. Why wasn't the yoga solving these problems? I felt as though the yoga was keeping my head above water, but my lifestyle kept pushing me back in again.

Āyurveda, translated as the 'knowledge of life', gave me a framework for everything that came before it. Āyurveda generously offered a place for yoga, astrology, aromatherapy and psychotherapy alike. All were welcomed and all were important components in the lustrous picture of health that it painted.

Āyurveda is described as a heavy-weight system. Heavy in a good way because it doesn't skim the surface. It is vast, deep and comprehensive. It takes years to understand and needs a devoted mind. In 2000, I devoted myself to another four years of study in this great art because I had faith in its message and its method.

Fast forwards almost 20 years, it occurred to me that most yoga practised today is actually for health reasons not spiritual ones. Classical yoga is devoted to helping the individual soul free itself from the shackles of mind/body consciousness and identify with the ocean of energy all around us instead.

But Āyurveda says that in order to do that, you need good healthy foundations. The spiritual road is rocky and fraught with difficulty. It is not advisable to do heavy-duty yoga practices if you are physically and emotionally unhealthy. According to legend, Āyurveda was a gift from the gods to save us from ourselves. It certainly felt that way for me. I spent much of my 20s and early 30s immersed in tantric practices that weren't doing me much good at all. I was very emotionally volatile and needed help, though I didn't really see that at the time.

Āyurveda put a stop to many things and helped me make a start on self-repair in a sustainable way. My āsana and prāṇāyāma practice transformed, my meditation changed and my daily routines became unrecognizable. My back pain has now largely subsided unless I overdo it, and depression, though a familiar neighbour, is no longer a permanent sitting tenant. I am so much more stable now than I ever was.

Why this book?

A lot of water has passed under the bridge since I started this adventure in my late teens.

But I've been around the block so many times now that if I don't start sharing my experiences and understanding, I'll soon forget it all. Learning is a funny business. Once you know something, you soon forget how you got there. Can you remember all the steps you took when you learned how to drive? Wisdom is a distillation of years of trial and error. This book is an opportunity to trace back those steps so that others on a similar path can tread more easily and avoid the pitfalls that I encountered.

I've always been a teacher. I've taught almost everything I ever learned. I've been teaching since I was 22. I've never really done anything else apart from work in McDonald's when I was a teen. So, this book is for teachers. Yoga teachers mainly, but any teacher in a similar field might find my experience useful. Teachers of Āyurveda might find this book helpful for filling in the gaps in their knowledge of yoga. Teachers in related fields like naturopathy, Chinese medicine or aromatherapy might also get a lot of good ideas from this book, but my main avatar is the yoga teacher.

There are a few books that discuss what yoga and Āyurveda have in common but a lot of them are based on theory. This book is based on practice. I have had a long time to try it all out and see if all that theory is actually true. Some of it is and some definitely isn't. I'll share some of my best stuff with you. Course-planning ideas, lesson plans, sequences, all that stuff that takes time and effort to work out. Well, I've done the hard work for you. You can put your feet up a while longer and then swan in to your yoga class with some ready-made lesson plans ready to go

I would have loved to get a book like this when I started integrating Āyurveda into my yoga teaching and into my life. When I started giving workshops to yoga practitioners in 2001, no one had even heard of Āyurveda. Now it can be found on many teacher training curriculums. How far we've come! This book will speed up the process and pave the way for new generations of teachers who will be teaching with an awareness of Āyurveda from the word go.

Chapter 1

INTRODUCTION

You are a yoga teacher now. People look to you for guidance, inspiration. It feels like quite a responsibility. Are you up to the job, or do you still feel like an imposter? I know I do sometimes. I have to face up to my flaws every day and as I get older, it feels as though things are getting harder not easier. It's not easy being me. I wonder if everyone feels that way deep down.

Maybe so many of us feel that way because we have mistakenly given ourselves the wrong label, or perhaps we should never have tried to label ourselves at all. Labels are convenient. They give others an idea of the contents, but if we start with the supposition that every molecule of ice is unique in its beauty and design, then does simply calling it ice do it justice? We are much greater than the sum of our parts, and identifying with our roles does not help our cause.

Let me share a little secret with you. There's no one there really. The *you* that you think is running the show doesn't really exist and yet there you are. The unique qualities that make you who you are appear, hang around for a while and then disappear again. There's nothing permanent about you. The *you* that you think is there isn't really. There's no one there. Life is enjoying being you and then you are gone, and life will enjoy being something else.

Let me share another secret with you. It doesn't help to know that there's no one there, because apparently there is. You look in the mirror and there you are. You have this body, this mind, this personality and a story in which you play your part. Never tell yourself that life doesn't matter, because the fire in you makes it matter. Your story is important. Your part was chosen carefully, so play it as well as you can.

There are rules, of course. None of us get them when we are young. We walk head first into trouble all the time. It's amazing how so many of us made it to adulthood at all. Such is the blessing of the great mother who carefully nurtures and protects her children. Āyurveda is like a good mum. She makes sure we eat properly, keep warm, exercise appropriately and, well, you know the rest. Even if our own mother never held us so well, if we look around, we realize that her spirit is holding us all the time. We don't get very far when we try to go it alone. Even when we are arrogant enough to think we are doing so, we get help anyway. If we really pay attention, we realize that not everything in life is random. There are little arrows everywhere nudging us forwards. All we have to do is adjust our perception. Twiddle our radio knobs until we find a non-local channel. It changes what we see and how we see it. Life is imbibed with symbolism. That means that not everything is what is seems. Our pea brains can't take it all in, so we need to work a bit harder to unwrap the truth of things and see the bigger picture.

Luckily, many have trodden the path of life before us and left clues behind. We don't need to start from the beginning. We just need to study and explore the ideas of those who came before us with an open heart.

Another important truth is that you can't help everybody. As a general rule, you are best placed to help others who are in or have come from a similar life experience to you, so I have decided to write this book for yoga teachers. I could have written a book for minority groups, I suppose, because I belong to so many of them, but I didn't. I didn't because if I only had money to buy one book to inspire me then it would be this one.

For me, living an Āyurvedic life is looking forward. I hope this book inspires you too. There's a lot of good stuff in it. Practical, philosophical and even perhaps political. As yoga teachers, we have a place in society, so making statements about the state of the world and the societies we live in should not be removed from the overall landscape. So many personal development books seem to ignore this subject on the assumption that we can somehow create our own world in a bubble. From my experience, you can't. You cannot change your life without becoming fully conscious of your place in it. How you feel about yourself is shaped by your ethnicity, class, family and cultural values as well as the general values and mores of your country.

This is the stuff of yoga. We are not just working with our bodies. We are also working, arguably more importantly, with our minds and hearts. We are all living with limiting thoughts and beliefs that dictate the choices we make throughout the day. The tools of yoga and Āyurveda are tried and tested ways of dealing with them.

We know they work, otherwise we would not have become yoga teachers. In this book I am going to present a powerful programme to you that will keep you and your students reeling with wonder for years to come. It's a high claim that I take no credit for, because all I am doing is relaying ideas and practices that have been around for millennia.

My claims are made on the back of thousands who have devoted their lives to the laboratory of spiritual progress, so thank them afterwards. In traditional ashram life, we used to chant the names of all the sages of yoga that came before as a thank you for passing down the perennial wisdom, so I shall do the same. I would like to thank the following people: Vasant Lad, who has generously committed to offering five-day intensives in the UK for over ten years now. My vision has certainly been shaped by him. David Frawley, who has written several illuminating books on yoga and Āyurveda and whose books I recommend on my courses. All the doctors and lecturers who shared their knowledge with us on the very first degree course in Āyurveda in the UK back in 2000. My friend and colleague Dr Cathy Mae Karelse, with whom I have had the privilege of working for several years and who has made the path less lonely. Sian O'Neill, my lovely editor, who gave me the opportunity to write this book and share my work with a larger number of people in her two previous books *Yoga Teaching Handbook*[1] and *Yoga Student Handbook.*[2]

What's in this book?

This book is based on a classical model. It is based on Swatmarama's vision of Haṭha yoga as written in the *Haṭha Yoga Pradīpikā* (HYP)

1 O'Neill, S. (2017). *Yoga Teaching Handbook*. London: Jessica Kingsley Publishers.
2 O'Neill, S. (2019). *Yoga Student Handbook*. London: Jessica Kingsley Publishers.

around 1450 CE. It is based on the idea that physical and mental wellbeing have to come first. We need to be strong to brave the path of classical yoga because the true yogic path is like walking on a razor's edge. In deeper yogic practices, we have to confront ourselves. It sounds straightforward, but anyone who has trodden the path of personal development will tell you that confronting inner demons, limiting beliefs, unresolved grief, anger, rejection, despair, sadness and so on takes a very brave heart. Most of us prefer to numb ourselves with tranquilizers like TV, alcohol, food, sex and the endless distractions that the internet is so good at providing. We try to get from one end to the other with as little distress and pain as possible; but with a little more support and encouragement, we feel empowered to do more, want more and be more. I want this book to be another one of those little beacons of help, because all of the information herein certainly helped me.

All pages marked with ⬇ can be photocopied and downloaded at www.jkp.com/catalogue/book/9781787755956

Basic principles of Āyurveda

We cannot get to the nitty gritty of practice without painting the foundations first. Āyurvedic principles draw upon all six Darśanas or philosophical systems of the *Vedas*. However, the most influential system is Sāṃkhya, as propounded by Kapila in the 7th century BCE. Sāṃkhya is like a tree of manifestation that starts from a state of undifferentiated oneness or Brahman and takes us all the way down to you and me. The concepts of Prakṛti and Puruṣa will be discussed, as well as the five elements, three doṣas, five senses, sense organs and motor organs. It is important to have some understanding of this model before we can talk about yoga practices.

Agni

I will also introduce this hugely important concept from the get-go because it is the most important idea that links Āyurveda with classical yoga. All of the practices in the *HYP* are based on it, from āsana practice all the way through to the subtle practices of kundalini yoga.

Āsana

Most people come into yoga through āsana practice. This is because it is not only the most relevant and useful yoga practice for us, but also an important preparation for the more subtle practices that come later. The *HYP* also recommends we start with āsana.

I will present āsana practice from an Āyurvedic perspective. This means I will put forward ideas on how to work with the three doṣas, five elements, 20 qualities or gunas, how to make appropriate adjustments to daily and seasonal cycles and how to work with marma points.

Daily and seasonal regimens

You will read repeatedly that Āyurveda is not a quick fix. In fact, it is more of a slow fix in the sense that we have to change our day-to-day lives if we want healing to last, because most of the time our un-wellness is caused by the way we live our lives. That means what, how and when we eat, how we exercise, how we work, how we relate to others and when we sleep. This is one of the most important things that Āyurveda can teach us and indeed what we can teach our students.

Course planning and lesson planning

When I am leafing through a book written for teachers, one of the first things I look for is tips on lesson planning and course planning. Yoga teaching can get quite tedious and repetitive after a while, so we start looking for a bit of inspiration. Well, I am confident that this chapter will provide enough teaching ideas to keep you busy for months, if not years. You can start experimenting in your own practice and then put a programme together for your students. Your teaching will get fuller, richer and more relevant.

Marma

Marmani (plural) are like mini pools of prāṇa, more sensitive than the surrounding tissue and very important for maintaining good prāṇic flow through the body. Marmani is akin to pressure points used in Chinese medicine, and having trained in both systems, I will share some useful applications with you from the Chinese system too.

I've always been attracted to subtle practices, and one way of deepening one's experience of āsana practice is to use marmani as points of focus. Most marmani used in yoga will be in the hands, feet, spine and other major joints. There are 108 marma points mentioned by Susruta,[3] but I will only be focusing on the ones that can easily be located without needing loads of anatomical knowledge.

Working with marma points will not only help to improve overall circulation but will also support the healing of imbalances. Incorporating marmani into āsana work is something I have largely developed myself because not a lot of work has been done on it so far. It is my hope that this chapter will spur on other teachers to do more research and find novel ways of building marma work into yoga practice.

Rasāyana

No book on yoga and Āyurveda would be complete without some exploration of Rasāyana or rejuvenation practices. Yogic literature is littered with promises on how to overcome old age and disease, so I will explain this approach and map out all the key techniques recommended by Āyurveda that are applicable.

Subtle practices

Subtle work can include a whole number of practices and mainly refers to tantric techniques.

---

3 Mitra, J. (1998). *Suśruta-saṃhitā: Sūtrasthāna*. Chapter XXV. Varanasi: Chowkhamba Sanskrit Series Office.

Subtle practices include the following:

- **Prāṇāyāma:** The expansion and control of prāṇa.
- **Mudrā and bandha:** The management and manipulation of prāṇa.
- **Chākras:** Visualization work, as well as concentration techniques on particular points along the spine and the front of the body.
- **Mindful breathing:** Using the breath itself as a focal point for attention during meditation and āsana work.

Yoga Nidrā

Everyone loves Yoga Nidrā. I think this is because we are all so tired. People work really hard, and then get little respite from their mind and senses because they swap one kind of stress for another. TV is not a legitimate form of relaxation, really. Regular Yoga Nidrā can deeply replenish us and our students because it goes deep. It is not meant to be a relaxation per se but ends up being so. It is a deeply therapeutic process that is actually quite hard work in its own right, but many people use it to zone out and get some deep rest, which is a welcome by-product of the process.

Mantra

I have devoted a few pages to mantra work because Āyurveda considers it to be the most important tool for working with the mind. Mantra work can be mind-boggling for western yoga teachers because most of us haven't studied much Sanskrit and our pronunciation is a bit rubbish, so I have limited most of the content to simple stuff like Bīja mantras (single-syllable mantras) that don't pose too much of a tongue-twisting challenge for yoga teachers.

Sanskrit terms

I won't lie. I use a lot of Sanskrit terms in this book. This is because I believe it is important to embrace the heritage from which both yoga and Āyurveda come. Sanskrit adds a layer of understanding that is deeper than the practice or the translated concept. There is power in the sounds of words themselves. I have tried to remain faithful to the academic protocol of using diacritics, to help you gain some idea of how it would sound in Sanskrit.

There are some simple rules. When there is a line above a vowel, like in *āsana*, the vowel is long (*aasana*). When there is an accent or a dot under or over s, like ś and ṣ, it is pronounced 'sh' as in 'shoe', so *Śīrṣāsana* should be pronounced *shirshasana*. Those are the key basics. The rest is rather complicated, and I recommend you do a short Sanskrit course if you really want to get to grips with it, but you really don't need it to gain from this book or to be a good yoga teacher.

Understanding Āyurvedic protocols

This book is mainly about helping you and your students get the best out of everyday life, but it is worth knowing that in the world of Āyurveda, deeper interventions are possible.

Proper Āyurvedic clinics offer profound and transformative treatments that can turn you inside out.

Āyurvedic health spas offer a wide range of therapeutic treatments that can be found in the more so-called serious clinics, but spas have a different goal. Spas generally offer treatments that promote wellbeing, whereas the deeper Āyurvedic treatments are a major intervention in many serious health conditions. It is important to understand this difference when you are looking for help.

Āyurveda approaches health imbalances in two fundamental ways:

- **Śamana Chikitsā:** This means 'pacifying treatment' or 'palliative treatment'. It involves all the things we generally associate with Āyurveda, like dietary changes, taking herbs, doing yoga and meditation and making changes to our behaviour and attitude in terms of the way we carry ourselves in the world. Most of this book will focus on Śamana Chikitsā.

- **Śodhana Chikitsā:** This means 'purifying treatment'. Āyurveda employs panchakarma or five-action treatment to help clear the body of exogenous toxins and endogenous imbalances caused by an excess build-up of the doṣas. The first part of panchakarma involves āma pāchana, or clearing the digestive tract of āma, toxicity. This is done with diet control and herbs. Thereafter, a practitioner will set up a treatment plan that prepares the client for one of the major treatments. The five treatments are as follows:

- **Vaṃana:** Inducing emesis to clear excess kapha from the body.
- **Virechana:** Prescribing appropriate purgatives to clear excess pitta from the body.
- **Basti:** The application of enema therapy to clear excess vāta from the body.
- **Nasya:** Applying herbal drops to the nose to help clear excess doṣas in the head and neck.
- **Rakta Mokṣana:** Bloodletting using either leeches or a syringe. This is believed to help clear toxins from the blood.

— *Chapter 2* —

HISTORY OF ĀYURVEDA FROM A YOGIC PERSPECTIVE

Āyurveda has been around forever.

Well, that's the common phrase we use when we mean 'a very long time'. But I mean 'literally forever', because Āyurveda is timeless. It means 'knowledge of life', which is kind of ironic because life has always known itself and we have always been a part of it, but our conscious minds are trying to fathom the great mystery. Our existence is a mystery to us and our understanding of our place in the universe is still in its infancy, but Āyurveda sends us a clear signal from the outset, and even though it seems like we are still grappling in the dark, given half the chance, the body can look after itself because it is plugged in to the whole.

But how old is old?

Like most things Indian, Āyurveda can be traced back to Vedic literature, which dates back to 6000 BCE. The four major Vedic works are:

- *Rig Veda*
- *Yajur Veda*
- *Sama Veda*

- *Atharvā Veda.*

Out of these four, the *Rig Veda* and the *Atharvā Veda* have contributed the most to building the foundations that became the edifice of Āyurveda.

The *Rig Veda* introduced many concepts that are still used in Āyurveda today. They include:

- The three doṣas (described as tridhātu, which means 'three tissues')
- Agni, the sacred god of fire
- Soma, the water god
- Key organs, common diseases and over a hundred herbs
- Healing mantras still commonly chanted today.

The *Atharvā Veda* is a major precursor to modern Āyurveda. *Atharvā* means 'medicine' and refers not only to herbs but also to mantra and japa (repetition of mantra). There are many references to all eight branches of Āyurveda, including internal medicine, gynaecology and obstetrics, longevity and virility (Rasāyana and Vājīkaraṇa), surgical procedures, eye diseases and poisoning. It mentions the three doṣas and agni as the key players in the digestion of food, and includes a detailed description of Āyurvedic anatomy and a long list of diseases, herbs and treatments.

Mythology

According to the *Caraka Saṃhitā*, which was redacted around 400 BCE, the teachings of Āyurveda were passed down from divine beginnings and developed into a system that mere mortals like us could understand and benefit from. The great creative god Brahma taught it to Daksha Prajapati, who taught it to the Ashwins (celestial twins), who taught it to Indra, who then apparently passed it down to a variety of sages. Indian mythology is complicated and not all that relevant to this work, so I'm keeping it brief. Suffice it to know that the great *Caraka Saṃhitā* is a summary of the teachings of one lineage of teaching and the *Suśruta Saṃhitā*, another lineage. Charaka was really hot on philosophy, so the fundamental principles taught today are based on his understanding. Susruta was a surgeon, so a lot of the technical stuff used today is inspired by him, including the use of marma points, which I will be covering in this book.

Other references

It's worth mentioning that aspects of Āyurveda were also mentioned in the Indian epic *Mahabharata* (900 BCE), the teachings of Buddha (500 BCE), the *Ramayana* (300 BCE) and the *Upaniṣads* (many works spanning over a thousand years). In other words, Āyurveda pretty much got everywhere and has been around forever!

Classical texts of Āyurveda

The three major compilations that form the backbone of Āyurveda are:

- *Caraka Saṃhitā*
- *Suśruta Saṃhitā*
- *Aṣṭāṅga Saṅgraha.*

They are known as the Brihat-trayi, the great triad, and were written in Sanskrit verses known as slokas.

Caraka Saṃhitā is the most well known and influential. It was thought to have been written between the Panini period and King Kanishka's rule, which puts it around the 2nd century BCE. The current format of *Caraka Saṃhitā* was not completed until around the 4th century as more information came to light. It is made up of eight sections known as sthānas. Most of the fundamental principles are presented in the first and biggest section, the *Sūtrasthāna*, which has 30 chapters.

The eight sections deal with all the key clinical areas of Āyurveda, which are:

- Kāyacikitsā (general medicine)
- Balachikitsā (obstectrics/paediatrics)
- Graha Chikitsā (psychiatry)
- Śalyatantra Chikitsā (surgery)

- Śālākyatantra Chikitsā (ear, nose and throat (ENT) and cephalic diseases)
- Viṣa Chikitsā (toxicology)
- Rasāyana (rejuvenation therapy)
- Vājīkaraṇa (treatment for improving libido).

Caraka Saṃhitā makes references to certain surgical procedures (Shalya Tantra) mentioned in the *Suśruta Saṃhitā*, which suggests that the latter is older, although the compilation in its current form was written after the *Caraka Saṃhitā*. Susruta was a well-known surgeon who performed the first rhinoplasty and also detailed the locations of 107 marma points. *Suśruta Saṃhitā* is structured in a similar way to *Caraka Saṃhitā*.

Aṣṭāṅga Saṅgraha was written by Vagbhata around 400 CE. It is more elaborate in its explanations than its cousins but is similar in structure.

Aṣṭāṅga Hṛdaya was written around the same time by a different Vagbhata in southern India. It is a more precisely edited version of the *Aṣṭāṅga Saṅgraha* and is widely used as a reference text in the Āyurvedic community even today. The verses are more poetic and easier to memorize and many modern Indian Āyurvedic physicians know it by heart.

Āyurveda and Haṭha yoga

Yoga and Āyurveda as sister sciences

Many modern yoga texts refer to yoga and Āyurveda as sister sciences and this is a very useful analogy because they have a common vision and can be logically amalgamated into a continuum of development that is mutually complementary. It is important to recognize, however, that the strength of these links is a modern appropriation that does not necessarily have as much literary support as we would like to think.

The pre-scientific medical paradigm of India was based on a holistic approach that came to be systematized into the main corpus of Āyurveda,[1] but many of the medical references made in classical yoga texts actually predated Āyurveda and came from the tantras. This means that Āyurveda

1 *Caraka Saṃhitā, Suśruta Saṃhitā* and *Aṣṭāṅga Hṛdaya*.

is not the only medical reference point, but it is certainly a major player because it is the only system that makes concepts like the doṣas, vāta, pitta, kapha, the dhātus *et al.* meaningful. The *Caraka Saṃhitā* fleshes out these concepts and presents them in the broader holistic context of the Sanātana Dharma[2] (eternal truth) as laid out in Vedic literature.

Most of the main literary and cultural influences of India of old existed within the Vedic landscape. Each work has its own specialism. Classical yoga texts focus on the goal of enlightenment and the techniques to achieve it but make generalized references to the medical benefits of those techniques. Jason Birch points out, for example, that when an āsana or a prāṇāyāma practice is said to cure all diseases, this is more to do with literary style than clinical observation.[3]

In other words, it is important not to take these statements too literally or ponder over their validity. The broad-sweep approach to these statements is a strong indication that the writers of yoga texts[4] were not medical experts but were rather looking to galvanize enthusiasm for their techniques.

If we are to accept that classical yoga belongs to this pre-scientific view of the body, then it stands to reason that we should try to build on this paradigm and apply it to the way we use yoga today. Building bridges between the two systems can only enhance our overall understanding, not detract from it.

By understanding the general tenets of this ancient medical model, we can learn to articulate our experiences of yoga practices using traditional terms and further substantiate the Vedic paradigm.

Haṭha Yoga Pradīpikā

In the *HYP*, Swatmarama borrows many ideas from the tantras as well as Āyurveda to flesh out his system of yoga. His generalizations suggest that

2 Yogapedia (2018). *Sanātana Dharma.* Accessed on 18/2/2021 at www.yogapedia.com/definition/6240/Sanātana-dharma.

3 Birch, J. (2018). Pre-modern Yoga Traditions and Āyurveda: Preliminary Remarks on Shared Terminology, Theory and Praxis. School of Oriental and African Studies. London University. Accessed on 1/3/21 at http://hssa-journal.org.

4 *Vasisthasamhita* (12–13th century); *Yogataravali* (14th century); *Gorakshasataka* (13–14th century); *Yogayajñāvalkya* (13–14th century); *Sivasamhita* (15th century).

he may not have been an Āyurvedic expert, but his methods fit in very well with the vision that both yoga and Āyurveda share.

Common visions

David Frawley[5] delineates the thin line that differentiates the primary goals of yoga and Āyurveda. He explains that yoga is first and foremost a science for self-realization, and Āyurveda is mainly the science of self-healing. This is useful because if we adopt this idea, we come to realize that the yoga we practise today is more aligned with the goals of Āyurveda than it is with classical yoga. Yoga is generally practised for its physical and emotional health benefits rather than as a tool for spiritual liberation.

This is right and proper because any attempt to jump ahead and practise the deeper tantric techniques hinted at in the *HYP* would be unlikely to reap results at best and could be damaging at worst. We are warned that we cannot expect to run before we can walk.

The pathway set out by the *HYP* is a sensible approach that can only be fully understood once we understand the basic principles of Āyurveda.

Purification

The model of yoga taught in the *HYP* is based on the concept of purification (Śodhana). This idea must be applied to the overall medical paradigm from which both yoga and Āyurveda grew. We cannot assess these ideas from a modern perspective, nor can we ever understand why the pathway was laid out as such, unless we understand the basics of Āyurveda.

Agni

One of the key concepts that bridge yoga and Āyurveda is the idea of agni.

Agni, meaning 'fire', was adopted by both systems of Āyurveda and yoga but actually originates from the *Rig Veda* in which it was worshipped as a deity.

5 Frawley, D. (1999). *Yoga and Āyurveda*. Twin Lakes, WI: Lotus Press.

Agni is a key metaphor for measuring the quality of one's health and wellbeing and in the *HYP* is a key tool for both purification and transformation. It is generally translated as digestive fire, but it has a broader remit than this.

Swatmarama uses the same physiological principles as Āyurveda to map the Haṭha yoga process. The quality of one's physical health is reflected in the strength of one's agni, which moves from purification of the physical body to the prāṇic body. It is the main measuring tool for assessing our preparedness for the various stages of Haṭha yoga practice. It also is the main catalyst for galvanizing the awakening of kundalini shakti.

Swatmarama's Haṭha yoga

The process of development laid out by Swatmarama is summarized in the first verse:

> Salutations to the glorious primal guru, Sri Ādinātha who instructed the knowledge of Haṭha yoga which shines forth as a stairway for those who wish to ascend the highest stage of yoga, raja yoga.[6]

Raja yoga refers to Patanjali's *Yoga Sutras*, written around 1500 years earlier. From this verse, we can infer that Haṭha yoga is an effective means of fulfilling the goals of raja yoga, which would otherwise be unachievable for most.

Before revealing any techniques, Swatmarama takes some time to lay the foundations.

First, he identifies issues pertaining to attitude and mind. He highlights the key reasons why students fail and the ingredients needed for their success.[7] He soon follows this with an expanded version of Patanjali's Yama and Niyama.[8] Unlike Patanjali, however, Swatmarama spends relatively little time discussing the role of mind.

6 Muktibodhananda, Swami (1998). *Haṭha Yoga Pradīpikā.* (Third edition.) Bihar: Yoga Publications Trust. Chapter 1, Verse 1.

7 *Ibid.* Chapter 1, Verses 15 and 16 (i).

8 *Ibid.* Chapter 1, Verse 16 (ii, iii).

Why is it useful for yoga teachers to know about the Haṭha Yoga Pradīpikā?

Swatmarama may not necessarily have been an expert in Āyurveda; however, the HYP builds very compelling bridges between the two practices. Taking the two bodies of knowledge together presents a much richer landscape of the culture and values of ancient India from which they both flourished.

How we instruct

Many yoga teachers use a mishmash of instructions that include some science with a peppering of exaggerated claims borrowed from classical teachings. Unfortunately, this ends up being messy because we do not understand the science well enough to substantiate what we say, nor do we understand the thinking behind the claims made in classical texts like the *HYP*. Learning about the fundamental principles of Āyurveda gives us a firm footing in the latter. An understanding of Āyurvedic physiology helps us to plan better classes in classical yoga and teach with more congruence.

It is important to choose the basis on which you want to teach and to have a primary point of reference that is supported by other points of view. It is best to teach by one fully developed model than several half-baked ones. When I teach, I mainly refer to the Āyurvedic world view of doṣas, winds, heat, gunas, dhātus, agni and so on. I sometimes use scientific language to support my ideas, but my teachings remain consistent with a single world view. You need to decide and go with what inspires you.

The *HYP* adheres to this classical view, and the system it lays out is a progressive practice that prepares you for tantric meditation.

Here is the *HYP* pathway:

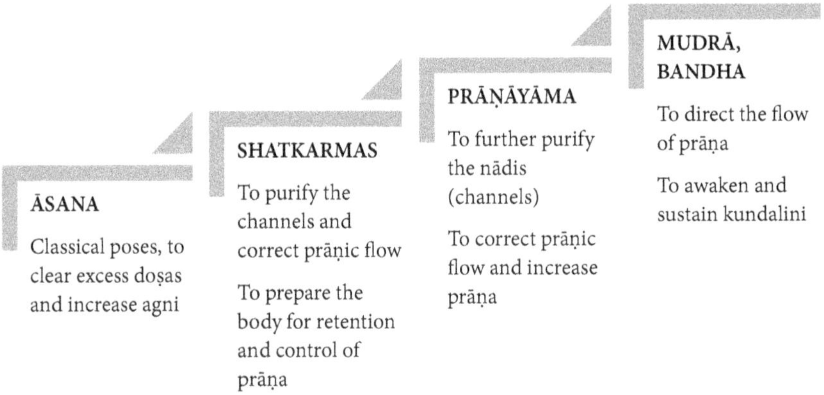

ĀSANA
Classical poses, to clear excess doṣas and increase agni
SHATKARMAS
To purify the channels and correct prāṇic flow
To prepare the body for retention and control of prāṇa
PRĀṆĀYĀMA
To further purify the nādis (channels)
To correct prāṇic flow and increase prāṇa
MUDRĀ, BANDHA
To direct the flow of prāṇa
To awaken and sustain kundalini

Figure 2.1: The *Haṭha Yoga Pradīpikā* Pathway

Many of the techniques of Haṭha yoga that we take for granted today refer to the same physiology and use the same language as Āyurveda, which is why a deeper understanding of Āyurveda can help us paint a fuller picture for our students.

— Chapter 3 —

PRAKṚTI: WHAT YOU WERE DESIGNED TO BECOME

The concept of self-identity is blurry. We think we know who we are, but our sense of self evolves as we mature and age. A more evolved version of oneself can look back and identify qualities that have always been there. These constant qualities give us a clue about the essence of our nature. Essential qualities are not linked to good or bad behaviour. A good upbringing can bring out the best in us and a bad one the worst. A warped oak tree that has been battered by storms, pollution and infection is still essentially an oak tree. The warped tree is in a state of Vikṛti. It has tried its best to remain robust and become what was intended but it has had to adapt itself heavily to unfavourable conditions, ending up a lesser version of what it could have been. A twisted, stunted tree, however, is still beautiful and perfect in its own right.

It is important to learn how to differentiate between how we turned out and our essential nature. Most of us can be more than what we are if our life conditions change. Like the oak tree, we can be better versions of ourselves with the right amount of sun, water and nutrients. We must be careful not to over-identify with flaws and assume they are part and parcel of who we are.

Not identifying does not mean denying. Accepting what we have become is important to cultivating a more generous and forgiving mindset.

Seeing ourselves as constantly lacking only perpetuates discontentment because we are never complete. A mind that sees lack and imperfection always will, even if it is no longer true. The glass can never be seen as half full, because we are in the habit of seeing the opposite. It is better to view a cracked pot as something that can be made beautiful by filling the cracks with gold, as the Japanese used to do.

The relationship between our essential nature (Prakṛti) and the imperfect yet still lovable version of ourselves that we become (Vikṛti) is a dynamic one. There is always wholeness yet this wholeness is in a constant state of flux, so we find ourselves moving in and out of kilter like an elastic band, towards and away from a state of homoeostasis. With strong foundations and an awareness of our essential nature, periods of imbalance are shorter. We recover from illness more quickly and spring back from emotional upsets without lasting damage.

Prakṛti and Puruṣa

Before we explore prakṛti with a small p in more depth, let us take a moment to consider Prakṛti with a big P. In the wider context of Sāṃkhya philosophy, the machinations of the cosmos are explained in 24 parts.

Consciousness is essentially undifferentiated oneness (Brahman) that becomes two: the manifest universe (Prakṛti) and the retained consciousness that underpins it (Puruṣa). All that is observable as well as latent in the field of mother nature is Prakṛti and everything born into Prakṛti has senses, a mind and a separate body made up of the five elements that function as the three doṣas. Puruṣa is passive and can be likened to the 'Infinite-I' also known as the 'Higher-Self' or 'God-Consciousness'. The term Ātman is used in many great works of Indian literature and is conceptually similar. Puruṣa is not part of the field of Prakṛti so is not knowable by the lower mind or manas. It can be known by our wisdom mind or buddhi, which is not driven by our ego: instincts. Puruṣa underpins everything because without it there can be no consciousness or awareness. When we open our eyes, god looks out through them. We only think we are separate because of our innate instinct for self-protection, but this self-protective mechanism is not who we really are. The dynamic field of life belongs to Prakṛti; but without Puruṣa, Prakṛti remains unconscious.

Āyurveda and the self

Āyurveda applies the term Prakṛti to our own unique nature. In this sense, our unique Prakṛti is a fragment of the whole. We are an expression of the qualities and conditions that arose at a particular moment in time at a particular location. Every moment is unique and everything that is born of any given moment embodies the qualities of that moment. Every species in every land will be influenced by the characteristics of a particular moment in time, but that particularity is superseded by environmental and biological factors.

When we look at a nature close up, we can see that pretty much everything created has a unique nature. Slugs are slow and slimy, birds are light and fast, elephants are slow and bulky and so on. At the same time, everything is interdependent. We are realizing that we are part of a much larger community of life and cannot survive in isolation. Even our own body could be seen as a complex ecosystem in itself. We house billions of bacteria and viruses that form part of us, so *I* as a subject is always a *we*, a collective. Our sense of separateness is, therefore, not really true but rather more of a collective, a community of beings that work together as a whole.

Why is it important to know your Prakṛti?

In some respects, it isn't important at all. We don't have to be able to articulate who we are to be happy. We encounter our preferences as we go through life and value experiences that match our particular point of view at that time. We learn about what we like and what we don't and build attachments to those preferences. Our Prakṛti takes shape and by the time we are 30, we have become conscious of most facets of ourselves.

The astrological matrix

The idea that we are an expression of all the qualities that arose in a particular moment in time and space seems very abstract, but the model is profound and has been adapted by many modern schools of thought, in particular, Jungian and Transpersonal psychotherapy.

The astrological paradigm is truly holistic but very specific. It is based on the Law of Correspondences,[1] which means that what appears to be apparently separate actually belongs to a symbolic family that shares a similar resonance.

Why a yoga teacher should understand Prakṛti

Understanding how to pick up typical behavioural characteristics of common prakṛtis in your classes will make you a better teacher, but that is not the only reason or even the most important one. One thing that is often overlooked is that a good teacher teaches from the heart. When you become more conscious of your own behaviour, you will be better placed to understand your relationship with yoga, which in turn will help you bring out the best in yourself and inspire your students. You can encourage your students to follow a similar approach.

There is a hidden matrix that draws people together, so have faith that you will find your niche. A student should be inspired by you in some way. Inspiration is Nature's way of saying there is resonance. If a yoga teacher leaves you cold, move on. If a yoga student is not benefiting from your teaching, encourage them to move on too. Don't just hang on to them. You are doing them a disservice.

Prakṛti and Dharma

Dharma is an important concept in Vedic thought and refers to our sense of place in society, what we are able to contribute and our role in the community. Through experience, we become aware of what we have a natural aptitude for. We may be good with numbers, for example, or perhaps we are the more practical type. This ability helps us to create positive action so that we may serve others and find our vocation. If we are lucky, we will also find our work fulfilling, but this is not necessarily so. The rewards may be reaped elsewhere depending on the yearnings of our soul. It is important to consider this because if we do not sit comfortably in our social role, this will impact on our health and wellbeing. Dharma should

1 Three Initiates. (2018). *The Kybalion, Hermetic Philosophy*. UK: Perennial Press.

be a way of honouring our prakṛti in the way we serve others. Our place in society may be very humble or we may end up moving mountains. It doesn't matter. It is much better to be a happy care worker than an unhappy CEO. Does yoga teaching bring out the best in you?

Āyurvedic Prakṛti

The *Caraka Saṃhitā*[2] outlines a unique perspective on prakṛti.

Parental doṣas during the time of conception

Charaka says that the dominant doṣas in both parents during the time of conception determine the predominant doṣas the child will be born with. For example, if at the time of conception, the mother is feeling very kapha and the father very pitta, this combination will create a bidoshic pitta-kapha child.

Genetic and congenital factors

Our genes provide an important framework that explains why we turn out the way we do. We are made from the flesh and blood of our parents and carry a lot of their genetic material. This is hugely important and an inevitable factor in prakṛti, but it is wrong to think that it is the only factor. Genes can be switched on and off according to lifestyle factors, so we are not automatically disposed to suffer from genetic diseases.

Karma and the soul

The Ātman or the transmigrating soul is the true essence of our unique constitution. According to the *Vedas*, we are not just a conglomeration of genetic material that responds to external factors – environmental, astrological or otherwise. Āyurveda assumes that the pearl of existence is

2 Sharma, P.V. (2000). *Caraka-saṃhitā*. (Sixth edition.) Varanasi: Chaukhambha Orientalia. (p.337)

the soul, which can live through thousands of lifetimes before re-merging with oneness.

When we talk of the spiritual journey, this is the journey of the soul. A young soul is said to be hungry for new experiences, and an old soul is moving ever closer to reuniting with oneness where separate consciousness is no longer desired. Prakṛti is the garb that the soul has assumed, so at first it may take some time for our soul to acquaint itself with its new body and mind. We find out who we are by living.

Some people become conscious of assets gained from previous lives very quickly. Mozart, for example, could play the piano by the age of four. Good parenting can help a child recognize their innate strengths and weaknesses and harness them. We inherit behavioural tendencies too but with the right resources, we may be able to do better with them than our ancestors did.

Our doshic Prakṛti

Charaka lists all the possible combinations that are possible in the formation of the Āyurvedic prakṛti.

TABLE 3.1: THE SEVEN DOSHIC PRAKṚTIS

Doṣas prakṛti combinations	Common characteristics
Vāta	Light and dry. Sensitive.
Pitta	Hot and driven. Passionate.
Kapha	Heavyset. Slow and caring.
Vāta pitta	Light, active, driven.
Vāta kapha	Mentally lighter, physically heavier.
Pitta kapha	Hard working. Ambitious.
Vāta pitta kapha	Versatile and moderate.

Prakṛti is like a hologram

The manifest universe is not as solid as we might think. Under a microscope, it is mostly empty space, and many quantum physicists as well as mystics believe that everything that arises in the manifest world has the fleeting quality of dreams. A hologram can be seen as an analogy for Prakṛti: a hologram is the projection of a three-dimensional image that originates from somewhere else; that 'somewhere else' is the cosmic soup of infinite possibility or Brahman. Everything that arises in Prakṛti is a pattern of frequencies or waves that condense or collapse into particles of matter, and what ends up as solid depends on which waves our mind is attuned to (like a radio) and able to convert into an experience.

We are therefore living in a subjective universe, a hologram of our own soul's making. What we experience in our everyday life is a limited set of frequencies that have condensed as a result of the coming together of certain conditions at a certain time and place.

There is a hidden architect beyond our conscious field of awareness. Davies[3] believes that our lower mind only has the capacity to 'perceive' what has already been decided for us by our Higher-Self or Infinite-I, so we have less control over our lives than we think. Our mind is like an antenna that picks up information that is sent from outside our field of awareness, so the only thing we have agency over is how we *react* to what life brings us. If this is true, we can heave a sigh of relief and relax a little more often. Our soul or Ātman is in the driving seat and we are in the back seat taking it all in. We can make special requests and we may or may not get what we want because we are not the true driver.

It is not possible to prove this hypothesis one way or the other, but it is important to at least acknowledge that this existential debate continues to rage on. These big questions were debated in the *Caraka Saṃhitā* 2000 years ago and will continue far into the future as more and more information about the nature of reality comes to light.

3 Davies, S. (2010). *Butterflies are Free to Fly*. USA: L&G Productions LLC.

— *Chapter 4* —

FIVE ELEMENTS AND THREE DOṢAS

The Vedic vision of life is truly awe-inspiring. It speaks of unimaginable periods of time and powerful forces that shift, transform and interact. The essence of life and the true nature of all things is Sat-Chit-Ananda: existence, consciousness and bliss, the primary expressions of Brahman, the ultimate reality. Our Ātman or soul is endowed with the three powers of Sacchidānanda. These are:

- Life (Jiva)
- Light (Jyoti)
- Love (Prema).[1]

These three forces gradually condense into the world of matter that we experience through our senses and sense organs.

Matter is made up of the five elements (earth, water, fire, air and space), which are utilized by the three essences (prāṇa, tejas and ojas), which ultimately manifest into the three doṣas (vāta, pitta and kapha).

1 Frawley, D. (1999). *Yoga and Āyurveda*. Twin Lakes, WI: Lotus Press. (p.70)

Panchamahabhutas: the five great elements

There are two ways of viewing the five elements. Earth is the heaviest and densest, so it has the most latent energy. However, if we look at matter under a microscope, matter is not as solid as we think. It is actually mainly made up of empty space, so from this point of view, the second pyramid in Figure 4.1 may be more accurate.

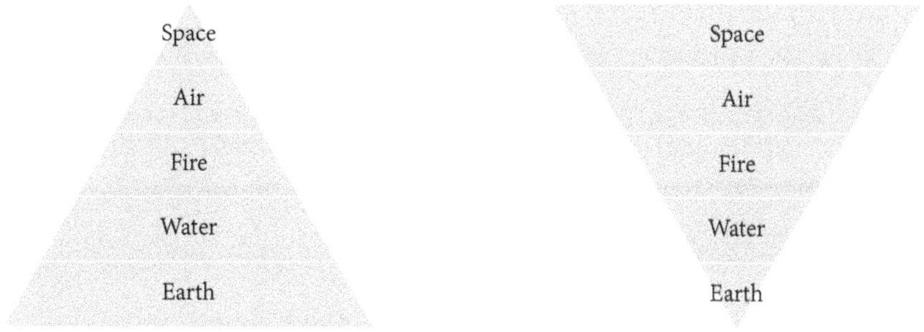

Figure 4.1: The Five Great Element Pyramid

It is important to note that the five elements are not literal. They are more symbolic in the sense of substances being more 'earth-like' or 'water-like' and so on. We experience the five elements by the qualities or gunas they possess. Āyurveda has listed 20 key qualities that form the spectrum of experience across the five elements.

TABLE 4.1: THE 20 ĀYURVEDIC GUNAS

Sanskrit	English	English	Sanskrit
Guru	Heavy	Light	Laghu
Manda	Slow/dull	Quick/sharp	Tīkṣṇa
Śīta	Cold	Hot	Uṣṇa
Snigdha	Oily (unctuous)	Dry	Rūkṣa
Slakshna	Smooth	Rough	Khara
Sāndra	Solid	Liquid	Drava
Mṛdu	Soft	Hard	Kaṭhina
Sthira	Stable	Mobile	Chala
Sūkṣma	Subtle	Gross	Sthūla
Viśada	Clear	Slimy	Piccila

Our experience of the gunas is relative to our unique prakṛti in the sense that although we have a general consensus of what effect extreme experiences have on us, our actual perception of matter can vary slightly depending on how our prakṛti is put together.

We don't all experience the world in quite the same way, because we are wired differently. Understanding the gunas is essential to understanding why and how we are different from each other and why we need to cultivate tolerance and cooperation in order to work together.

First, we need to consider which gunas apply to which elements and then apply those gunas to our experience of the world and of each other.

These traits also indicate the archetypal expressions of the 12 star signs. Space was not used in traditional astrology but integrates well with many of the characteristics of air.

TABLE 4.2: HOW TO WORK WITH THE FIVE ELEMENTS

	Earth	Water	Fire	Air	Space
Gunas/ qualities	Heavy Slow Cold Solid Stable Gross Hard	Cold Subtle Liquid Mobile	Subtle Light Sharp Hot Mobile	Cold Subtle Clear Light Dry	Subtle Clear
Nature	The ground beneath our feet Old trees with thick trunks Mountains Forests Elephants	Ocean River Rain Tsunami Stream Lake Well Jet Waterfall	Sun Fire Heat Light Lions Tigers Forest fires	Wind Hurricane Tornado Birds Mice Insects	Openness Desert Space Sky Atmosphere

Positive human traits	Down to earth Reliable Pragmatic Realist Hard working Loyal Tactile	Deep Adaptable Sensitive Emotional Creative Dreamy Healing	Passionate Driven Light up a room Positive Warm Generous Adventurous Sociable	Light Breezy Versatile Sociable Quick learner Commu-nicative Quick witted Rational Cool	Detached Hold others well Objective Cool Visionary
Negative human traits	Stubborn Heavy Stuck in a rut Fearful of change Lazy Hoarder	Wishy washy All at sea Unable to pin down Emotive Clingy Irrational	Angry Judgemental Demanding Intense Bossy Exhausting Impatient	Ungrounded Flighty Unstable Neurotic Anxious Confused Dry and cold	Heartless Cold Passive Unstable
Astrological sign	Taurus Virgo Capricorn	Cancer Scorpio Pisces	Aries Leo Sagittarius	Gemini Libra Aquarius	None

The three doṣas

The word 'doṣa' means 'fault', or 'disorder' and is thus named because we only really notice doṣas when we start to go out of balance. Doṣas reflect the temporary and ever-changing nature of Prakṛti as mother nature. Nothing remains the same for very long, but the rates of change can vary depending on the density of a bodily tissue. Bone, the densest tissue in the body, for example, replaces itself every seven years or so, but the stomach renews its lining every three days. Red blood cells are renewed every four months and so on.

There is a pattern that is copied every time tissues renew themselves and this pattern is based on the previous set of instructions rather than the original, which is why a scar can remain for life even though the skin renews itself regularly. It is incumbent on us to accept that change is the only constant. Our bodies are not designed to last forever, but we try our level best to maintain homoeostasis for as long as possible.

The doṣas represent the primary functions of the body that are needed to sustain and support life. These functional entities or forces are created when the five elements team up to fulfil specific purposes.

Kapha

Ka is one of the names of Brahma, the creative god. Some of its many meanings are 'body', 'sun', 'soul', 'water' and 'pleasure', which are all symbolically related. Pha means 'increasing' or 'flourishing', so we have the image of a body that is flush with life-giving water, a useful image to consider as we delve more deeply into the meaning of kapha.[2] As a whole word, 'kapha' means 'phlegm' or 'mucus', which is the main agent of lubrication in the body.

Earth and water work together to create a self-contained body. Our body is mainly made up of water, hence the term 'bag of water'. Kapha is tasked with building the body and keeping it hydrated and lubricated. Phlegm can be likened to the 'glue' that holds all the tissues together.

Kapha has a magnetic quality. Energetically, it is driven by the binding force of love. People who love each other stick together. It is the same with the body. Our bodies are like ecosystems where multiple organisms collaborate to create a single sense of belonging. Kapha resonates with the love of the soul (Prema) that makes us want to live. People who embody a lot of kapha energy tend to have a great capacity for love and compassion and this is reflected in their Dharma or social role.

Ojas is the essence of kapha, the vital juice that feeds our cells. When we have good ojas, our immune function is strong and we feel we have more endurance.

2 Wisdom Library (2020). *Kapha*. Accessed on 18/2/2021 at www.wisdomlib.org/definition/ka.

Kapha and the dhātus (tissues)

Kapha has a resonance with some bodily tissues more than others. It has a particular affinity with fat, possibly because like kapha itself, fat is stored fuel or potential energy. Kapha is inclined to hoard resources and this can often be seen in people who portray kapha qualities. Another word for 'fat' is 'snigdha', which also means 'loving and affectionate'.[3] The beauty of Sanskrit is that every word has a philosophical root that helps us understand its divine essence.

Kapha also has an affinity with rasa dhātu, which we would call 'blood plasma' and 'lymph'. Rasa is the most important of all seven tissue types because it is responsible for providing good-quality nutrients to all the other tissues. If the quality of what we eat is poor, the quality of rasa will be poor and, ultimately, our tissues will suffer. The function of rasa is Prīṇana, which means 'satisfying' or 'gratifying'. When the quality of food is good and our agni is strong, our body is deeply satisfied because it is properly nourished.

Functions of kapha

In general, kapha controls all anabolic processes. For this reason, it is very active during childhood, because children, by their very nature, are continuously growing. Babies are said to be like 'little bundles of joy' because they are full of Prema (bliss).

Kapha is responsible for hydration and lubrication and can be subdivided into five parts. The digestive tract is lined with mucus (kledaka kapha), which plays a vital part in providing an adequate fluid base for stomach acid and digestive juices to break down food and for food to pass along the tract smoothly through the rhythmic action of peristalsis.

The heart and lungs need adequate lubrication to remain properly nourished and to fulfil their vital functions (avalaṃbaka kapha).

The brain is suspended in a bag of fluid (cerebrospinal fluid), which is vital for nourishment and functioning not just of the brain, but of all the sense organs located in the head (tarpaka kapha). The word 'tarpaka'

3 Wisdom Library (2021). *Snigdha, Snigdhā*. Accessed on 18/2/2021 at www.wisdomlib.org/definition/snigdha.

means 'satisfying',[4] which provides a lot of clues to the nature of imbalances that may arise from lack.

Bodhaka kapha is located in the mouth in the form of saliva. The mouth is the doorway to nourishment and the instrument of love and affection, which are all kapha related. The word 'bodhaka' refers to both tongue and taste but also means 'informing', which touches on the idea of children using their taste buds to learn about new experiences and learning about things we have a 'taste' for.

We would not be able to move without the lubricating power of śleṣaka kapha in our joints. Śleṣaka means 'attaching' or 'connecting', so this kapha can be found in all the connecting parts, the major joints. Without kapha, moving would be impossible and, indeed, for many elderly people, the loss of joint lubrication causes a great deal of pain with movement.

The kapha type

Someone who expresses relatively high levels of kapha in their natural constitution usually has the following characteristics. See how many apply to you.

TABLE 4.3: THE KAPHA TYPE

Kapha	Tick
Physical characteristics	
Tall and sturdy, or short and stocky	
Heavy, solid build with lots of muscle and fat	
Round, soft contours to body	
Broad shoulders	
Thick neck	
Big hips	
Large joints	
Large, deep-set, watery eyes with thick eyelashes	

4 Wisdom Library (2021). *Tarpaka*. Accessed on 18/2/2021 at www.wisdomlib.org/definition/tarpaka.

Thick, oily skin that is often pale or white (relative to others in the same ethnic group)
Thick, wavy, lustrous hair
Large white teeth, strong gums and lush lips
Meaty calves
Deep, resonant voice
Large fleshy feet
Psychological traits
Calm, slow, cannot be rushed, good organizer
Good long-term memory but takes time to learn
Steady beliefs that don't change easily, stubborn
Greedy and possessive tendencies
Caring nature
Steady and regular, can get stuck in a rut
Likes to be practical
Slow and quiet
Cool, calm, uneventful
Sensitive to the touch and smell of others
Metabolic tendencies
Regular periods
Bowel movement may sometimes be prone to stickiness (mucus)
Sweat is cold with a pleasant smell
Appetite is regular, only needs one or two meals a day
Little thirst
Steady sexual desire, slow to get aroused, good endurance
Prone to heavy sleep
Prefers dry warm climates but generally not bothered
Strong immunity but prone to congestive disorders (mucus)
Normal circulation but can get sluggish with inadequate exercise
Total

Pitta

To support and sustain ourselves, we need an internal kitchen where food can be processed and used to nourish and support us. Every kitchen needs water and heat to prepare food. A good digestive system has just that. Our body uses water, acids, enzymes and bacteria to break down and distribute the food. This transformative process is called pitta, which is derived from the word 'tapas' meaning 'to heat'.[5] It is also often translated as 'bile' and can broadly be interpreted as that which *cooks*.

Water holds fire within it to protect the body from fire's destructive nature. We call this combination 'acid', and in the right portion, acid plays an essential role in breaking down food and transforming it into nutrients our body can use. It also plays a vital role in killing unwanted pathogens. There is stomach acid, which actually has a low pH in the lower part of the stomach only (1.0–4.0), but it is inaccurate to assume that all pitta locations are acidic. Every organ has its own optimal pH and, in fact, the seat of pitta, which is considered to be the small intestine, is more alkaline with a pH of 7.0–8.5.[6] The blood, also a pitta location, is alkaline at around 7.4, and the acidity can increase when there is poor oxygenation. The blood can build up unhealthy levels of carbon dioxide when respiration is inefficient, and this is one reason why blood can become more acidic. Imbalances in the pH can lead to pitta imbalances generally.

Tejas is the essence of pitta doṣa. The word has many meanings but in the Āyurvedic context it refers to some key attributes of fire expressed through the body. These include radiance, prowess, lustre, assertiveness and power. Tejas is strongly associated with the agni, the metabolic fire, which has similar attributes. This light ultimately originates from Jyoti, the divine light of Brahman.

Pitta and the dhātus

Āyurveda differentiates between red blood cells and blood plasma. Red blood cells are called rakta; blood plasma, which carries all nutrients

5 Wisdom Library (2021). *Pitta*. Accessed on 18/2/2021 at www.wisdomlib.org/definition/pitta.
6 News Medical (2018). *pH in the Human Body*. Accessed on 18/2/2021 at www.news-medical.net/health/pH-in-the-Human-Body.aspx.

around the body, is called rasa. Rakta is Jivana or life giving. Healthy blood is essential for good vitality.

Functions of pitta

Pitta controls all transformative functions in the body and mind and can be subdivided into five parts. In the digestive tract, pitta manages the digestion of food, which is the most important process for maintaining life. The word 'pachaka' means 'cooking' and as pāchakapitta is located in the seat of pitta, this is where it gets its meaning from.

Bhrājakapitta is located in the skin. The skin is the biggest organ in the body and is a kind of sheath between us and the outside world. The word 'bhrajaka' means 'make bright' or 'illuminate', so it is the light that we give off through our aura and complexion. It is the energy that lights up a room when bhrājakapitta is healthy. It also represents the heat we give off and the health of our blood.

There is a close association between bhrājakapitta and rañjaka pitta, which is located in the blood. Healthy blood is alkaline with ample red blood cells that are able to send prāṇa to the tissues. The liver is responsible for cleansing the blood, so rañjaka pitta is also associated with the liver. A sluggish or overworked liver will ultimately affect all pitta functions.

Ālocaka pitta is located in the eyes. For most people, the eyes are the most important organ for digesting impressions from the outside world.

Sādhakapitta represents the pitta energy that drives the mind. It controls the digestion of all impressions and information. People with strong sādhakapitta have very good critical and discriminative faculties. They are able to grasp ideas quickly and assess their validity.

The pitta type

Pitta types tend to be more visible than other doshic types because fire energy is naturally more 'out there'. Here are the common characteristics associated with pitta.

TABLE 4.4: THE PITTA TYPE

Pitta	Tick
Physical characteristics	
Medium, well-proportioned build (for your ethnicity)	
Soft, lustrous and warm skin, often freckled (depending on ethnicity), prone to acne or rashes when imbalanced	
Fine, soft and reddish hair (ethnically determined), men are often prone to early greying or balding	
Heart-shaped face, sharp contours	
Piercing eyes, intense gaze, eyes can get sore easily, sensitive to bright light	
Sharp tone to voice, concise use of language, impatient tone	
Psychological traits	
Precise, logical, good planner, sees things through, sharp	
Very good memory, quick to recall	
Very strong convictions, passionate, opinionated	
Prone to anger, judgemental, critical	
Intellectual, cerebral, goal oriented	
Ambitious, driven	
Argumentative	
Metabolic tendencies	
Profuse micturition, burning when unwell	
Loose, yellowish or burning stool when unwell	
Sweat copiously, strong fleshy smell	
Strong appetite	
Prone to excessive thirst	
Prefers cooler climates, easily irritated by heat and strong light	
Medium immunity, prone to infections, fevers and inflammation	
Strong circulation	
Pulse is wiry and jumpy, like a frog	
Total	

Vāta

Vāta manages all bodily functions including those of pitta and kapha. For this reason, it is called the 'master doṣa'. The word 'vāta' refers to the Vedic deity that presides over 'wind'. It can also mean 'wandering' and refer to the afflictions that it causes in the joints.

Wind is a very apt way of characterizing vāta because it is created by air moving through space. It has no physical substance but makes its presence felt by its functions and the impact it has on tissues.

Vāta originates from Jiva, that which brings life. It has no form other than vibration. It is a potential wave form that may be likened to sound in one sense but, in the quantum field, collapses into physical form when it matches with a particular frequency. Everything has a specific frequency, and this frequency is akin to its true nature. A radio can be seen as an analogy for this: on a radio you can only find a particular channel if you know its frequency; vāta holds this 'information' and needs it to engage with your cells. There is a lot of research currently taking place in the field of applied biophysics on the use of frequencies in medicine. Frequencies can have a powerful therapeutic impact on the body by amplifying cellular communication where it has been lost. Vāta, therefore, holds the secret behind the organizing frequencies of matter itself.

Vāta and the dhātus

Vāta has an affinity with the bones (asthi), which is kind of odd because bones are relatively hard and play a large part in our structure. Indeed, the main function according to Charaka is Dhāraṇā, which means 'support'. Asthi dhātu also provides the framework by which we move. The affinity between vāta and asthi is based on where vāta is felt when it is aggravated. When we get aches and pains, they tend to be in the joints of our back, neck, knees, hips and so on. When we get very cold, we feel the cold in our bones; and as we move into vāta age (post-menopause period), vāta can start to impact on the integrity of our bones when there is calcium loss. Vāta works with kapha to hold us together and keep us moving into old age. However, as we age, kapha reduces and vāta increases, so it becomes more important to manage the debilitating effects of vāta. This is the rationale as to why Charaka claims that kapha types tend to live longer.

Functions of vāta

Vāta controls all that moves in the body. This includes the following:

- Air that moves into the lungs via respiration
- Gases that move around the body via the bloodstream
- Food that moves along the digestive tract and the subsequent nutrients that are sent to the cells around the body
- Waste that moves out of the body, including urine, faeces and sweat
- Blood discharged in a woman's monthly cycle
- Information that moves from the brain, spinal cord and cells
- Information received from the senses and sent to the brain to be interpreted
- Motor functions
- Heart, circulation.

In fact, absolutely anything that involves movement of impressions, substances, solids or gases and even thought is controlled by vāta.

Charaka uses the word 'vayu' when describing the functions of the five sub-doṣas of vāta. It has exactly the same meaning as vāta but is used in slightly different contexts.

The five sub-doṣas or upadoṣas are mentioned in many yogic texts, as well as Āyurvedic ones. They are a way of rationalizing the electrical functions of the body, and opinions vary as to exactly what is attributed to what. I will try to keep the explanations relevant and useful.

PRĀṆA VAYU

Prāṇa vayu is located in the head and chest and is said to move inwards and downwards. In yogic texts, it is seated in the heart; but in Āyurveda, it is said to be seated in the head. In my opinion, it is both. When prāṇa enters the body through inhalation, it disperses into the head as well as the lungs. So even though the lungs pull it downwards via the action of the diaphragm, its presence remains in the head where it drives the mind and the senses. Prāṇa has a resonance with Anāhata Chākra and Ājñā Chākra.

From a classical point of view, the practice of Jālandhara bandha, or throat lock, is designed to encourage prāṇa to enter sushumna nādi and meet with apāna around Manipūra Chākra. Pratyahara, or withdrawal from the senses, prevents too much prāṇa from being used up by the mind and senses, thus making it more available to initiate a kundalini awakening.

The *Aṣṭāṅga Hṛdaya* summaries prāṇa vayu here:

> Prāṇa is located in the head and moves in the chest and throat. It supports the mind, heart, sense organs and intelligence. It attends to expectoration, sneezing, belching, inspiration and swallowing food.[7]

Here's what Vasant Lad says about prāṇa vayu:

> Prāṇa creates a union of outer cosmic prāṇa and inner prāṇa. Prāṇa is movement of mind, thoughts, feelings, emotions, sensation and perception. When prāṇa is motionless, it becomes blissful awareness.[8]

Prāṇāyāma means 'the controls and expansion of prāṇa'. Classical prāṇāyāma involves the retention of breath and this retention or kumbhaka can be as deeply satisfying as it can be energizing. It can also replenish a body and mind that is able to harness the prāṇa produced from it. Undigested prāṇa, however, can turn on the body and increase vāta, which is not desirable.

---

7 Murthy. S. (1999). *Vaghbata's Aṣṭāṅga Hṛdaya. Sūtrasthāna*. Varanasi: Krishnadas Academy. (p.167)

8 Lad, V. (2002). *Textbook of Āyurveda, Volume 1*. Albuquerque, NM: The Ayurvedic Press. (pp.48–53)

Here is a summary of the functions of prāṇa:

- Commands the buddhi (wisdom mind), heart and sense organs
- Helps push food down into stomach
- Salivation
- Sneezing
- Belching
- Breathing
- Stable functioning of nervous system
- Harnesses prāṇa from air and food to support and nourish the body.

UDĀNA VAYU

Udāna vayu is seated in the throat and moves upwards. The upward thrust of vāta originates in the diaphragm, so it is related to exhalation. It is the upward flow that nourishes the brain and also enables speech. Any āsana that encourages circulation toward the head could be said to promote udāna vayu (e.g., Adho Mukha Svanāsana (Downward Facing Dog pose)). Udāna vayu is an outward energy, so any energizing practice will also promote it. Udāna is associated with Vishuddhi Chākra in the throat.

Udāna vayu is often depleted after I have been teaching all day, so I go into 'mouna', which means 'silence'. I won't answer the phone or talk to anyone till the following day. People with hoarse voices tend to have depleted udāna vayu. According to the *Aṣṭāṅga Hṛdaya*,[9] udāna controls the following functions:

- Energy levels, strength and endurance
- The power to vocalize
- The capacity to memorise
- Skin complexion.

---

9 Murthy, S. (1999). *Vaghbata's Aṣṭāṅga Hṛdaya*. Sūtrasthāna. Varanasi: Krishnadas Academy. (p.167)

SAMĀNA VAYU

Samāna vayu controls the movement of the doṣas in the digestive tract. It controls secretions in all digestive organs, particularly the small intestine, liver and gall bladder. When samāna is functioning properly, both pāchakapitta (pitta in the small intestine) and kledaka kapha (kapha in the stomach) are able to function properly. Samāna is said to move from side to side, which is probably an interpretation of how food moves through the digestive tract. It is seated in the navel and is energetically controlled by Manipūra Chākra.

Here is what the *Aṣṭāṅga Hṛdaya* says about samāna:

> Samāna is located near agni, moves in the kostha (digestive tract) and holds food in the kostha while it cooks, separates out the essence from the waste and eliminates waste.[10]

Here is a summary of the key functions of samāna vayu:

- Reception of food
- Digestion of food
- Separating out food components and waste
- Sending waste downwards towards colon
- Providing strength and support to agni
- Supporting the doṣas in general
- Holding wastes (till they are ready to be excreted)
- Holding semen (till it is used)
- Holding menstrual fluid (till it is used).

APĀNA VAYU

Apāna vayu is seated in the colon and moves downwards. The primary seat of vāta is in the colon, so this makes apāna the most important vayu

10 *Ibid.*

to consider when assessing health. Apāna is associated with Svādishthāna Chākra and Mūlādhāra Chākra.

Apāna is also important in classical Haṭha yoga and relates to moola bandha. When moola bandha is engaged, this is meant to prevent apāna from being lost. Apāna is redirected upwards where it has the potential to engage with prāṇa around the area of Manipūra. This is one of the key goals of classical Haṭha yoga and the original aim of practising the bandhas (locks).

Here's what the *Aṣṭāṅga Hṛdaya* has to say about apāna:

> Apāna is located in the large intestines, moves in the waist, bladder, genitals and thighs and attends to the functions of elimination of semen, menstrual fluid, faeces, urine and the foetus.[11]

Vāta imbalances tend to start with dysfunctions related to apāna, so it is important to ensure proper functioning and flow before embarking on the practice of bandhas.

Here is a summary of the key functions of apāna vayu:

- Ejaculation of semen during sex
- Normal menstruation in women
- Proper and timely defecation
- Proper and timely voiding of urine
- Proper and timely delivery of child.

VYĀNA VAYU

Vyāna vayu is related to the general circulation, so it is seated in the heart. Any cardiovascular activity will relate to vyāna. Some of your students may get cold easily or experience cold hands and feet. Low circulation suggests that vyāna vayu needs close attention. Here is what the *Aṣṭāṅga Hṛdaya* says about vyāna:

> Vyāna is located in the heart, moves all over the body at great

11 *Ibid.*

> speed, attends to functions such as walking, bringing the body parts downwards, lifting the body parts upwards, opening and closing the eyes and so on. All mobility relates to vyāna.[12]

This statement means that all exercise and external movements of the body relate to vyāna. The other four vayus relate to internal functions, but vyāna is about how we move in the outer world. It is the first thing to go when we don't exercise sufficiently.

All five vayus are interrelated. Lifestyle may highlight a particular imbalance related to a single vayu; but left unattended, ultimately, all five vayus will go out of balance.

Vāta is the most important doṣa to take care of. Pitta and kapha cannot function healthily if vāta is unattended to. This is why yoga āsana is so useful for maintaining balance in the doṣas. Āsana is concerned with intelligent movement.

Here is a summary of the functions of vyāna vayu:

- Contraction and release of the heart muscle
- Distribution of rasa
- Upward and downward movement limbs
- Movement
- Food tasting
- Cleansing the channels
- Blood circulation
- Implantation and fertilization of ovum
- Separates metabolic wastes from food (helped by samāna vayu)
- Transports nutrients to tissues.

12 *Ibid.*

The vāta type

A vāta type is usually someone who is lightly built with fine features and prominent joints. There is a restless quality about vāta types akin to small active creatures like mice and birds. Vāta people have a lot of flair and can keep things light and fun when needed.

Here are the most common traits associated with vāta.

TABLE 4.5: THE VĀTA TYPE

Vāta	**Tick**
Physical traits	
Unusually short or tall	
Slight build, difficulty putting on weight	
Narrow hips and shoulders	
Prominent joints – often knobbly and cracking	
Difficulty putting on muscle	
Skin looks thin, dries, roughens and cracks easily, early wrinkles	
Hair is thin and coarse	
Face is long and angular	
Nose is often crooked	
Small, narrow, sunken, dark, dull, small eyelashes	
Teeth are often irregular with protruding and/or receding gums	
Lips are thin and narrow, dry easily	
Voice is often breathy and hoarse	
Psychological traits	
Superficial with many ideas, more thoughts than deeds	
Good short-term, poor long-term memory	
Frequently change their minds depending on mood, indecisive	
Fearful, anxious, insecure	
Prefer jobs that involve interacting with people and have varied activity	
Daily routines tend to be irregular and packed with activity, always on the go	
Very talkative and talk fast	
Sensitive to loud noises	
Metabolic tendencies	
Scanty, frequent micturition	

Bowel movement prone to variation, sometimes dry and hard, sometimes loose, frequent gas
Little sweat
Variable appetite, not that interested in food
Forgets to drink water or remain well hydrated
Quick to start but poor endurance
Quick to get sexually aroused, prone to overindulgence but with low endurance
Sleep is easily disturbed, prone to insomnia between 2am and 6am
Prefers warm weather at all times, loses strength in the winter
Weak immunity, gets sick easily
Prone to joint or back pain
Poor circulation, prone to cold hands and feet
Pulse is fast and slippery, like a snake
Total

Now check back and see which total is the highest.

If you have two doṣas that are very close in number, you are considered to be bidoshic. If all three doṣas are close in number, you are tridoshic. Charaka says that tridoshic types tend to have the strongest constitution, and those dominated by a single doṣa have the weakest. This is, however, a generalization and there are many other factors to consider.

I have amalgamated all three checklists in Appendix 1 for easy use with your students.

TABLE 4.6: THE FUNCTIONS OF THE SEVEN DHĀTUS

Dhātu	Tissues	Function
Rasa	Blood plasma and lymph	Prīṇana (gratifying)
Rakta	Red blood cells	Jivana (life giving)
Mamsa	Muscle	Lepa (covering)
Medas	Fat/adipose tissue	Snehana (oiling)
Asthi	Bone tissue	Dhāraṇā (supporting)
Majja	Bone marrow	Pūraṇa (filling: of bones)
Sukra/artava	Reproductive fluid (both sexes)	Garbhadhana (reproduction)

The three doṣas and the gunas

Now that we are familiar with the typical doshic types, we can summarize these traits using the Āyurvedic gunas. Charaka has attributed the following gunas and key characteristics to the three doṣas. He has listed a mixture of gunas and tastes (rasas).

TABLE 4.7: DOṢAS AND GUNAS

Vāta	Pitta	Kapha
Dry	Oily	Solid
Cold	Hot	Cold
Rough	Sharp	Smooth
Light	Light	Heavy
Mobile	Flowing	Stable
Irregular	Spreading	Sweet
	Sour	

The doṣas and time

TABLE 4.8: DOṢAS AND TIME

Vāta	Pitta	Kapha
2am–6am 2pm–6pm Brāhmamuhūrta (two muhurtas or 1 hour and 36 minutes before dawn) Dawn and dusk	10am–2pm 10pm–2am	6am–10am 6pm–10pm
Old age	Adulthood	Childhood
Late autumn and winter	Late spring and summer	Winter and early spring

The qualities of the doṣas may be amplified or pacified depending on the season, period of life and time of the day. For example, as vāta is light and mobile, it is better to wake up in the hours that lead up to dawn. If you wake up in kapha time, you may experience a heavier feeling and it will be harder to get up.

It is said that vāta controls old age because many of the diseases that are associated with old age are vāta in nature. Conversely, babies tend to experience diseases that produce more mucus.

The seasonal prevalence of gunas or qualities will depend on the country you live in, but it stands to reason that a hot season will eventually build up pitta doṣa, a cold, damp season will aggravate kapha doṣa and a cold, dry season will increase vāta doṣa.

Psychological gunas

Though the five elements also have psychological characteristics, Āyurveda draws upon the yogic gunas of tamas and rajas to explain the variation in attitudes that people live their lives by.

Tamas means 'darkness' or 'ignorance', so a tamasic mindset will be more likely to display the negative psychological traits of an element.

Rajas is characterized by a passion-driven mindset that seeks intense engagement with life. A rajasic mind is prone to constant emotional swings between pain and pleasure and is more likely to display the volatile qualities of the elements.

The lower analytical mind or manas is tasked with trying to make sense of the world as perceived by the five senses but it is not equipped to find its true nature. The only way the mind can settle is if we cultivate a third quality known as sattva, which is the quality of mind that is associated with clarity, harmony and balance. Sattva creates spaciousness and helps us control the negative impact of tamas and rajas.

Students in your class will display a variety of personality traits and physical characteristics. All students will be on a spectrum between the two extremes of the gunas. Some, for example, will be physically heavier and others lighter, some will be fast to learn and others slower, some will get hot easily and others get cold easily. When you are building a profile of each of your regular students, it is worth using the 20 gunas as a guide.

Students often confuse doshic mindsets with the psychological gunas. However, there is some co-relation between the character traits of each of the three doṣas and the three yogic gunas. For example, vāta or pitta types are more likely to have rajasic tendencies because of their restless nature. A kapha type is more likely to have tamasic tendencies because of kapha's tendency to stagnate.

That said, in your classes, you will also observe pitta students who may be depressed (tamasic pitta) and kapha students who may be anxious and restless (rajasic kapha) or angry and irritable (also rajasic kapha). You will also observe vāta students who are sometimes stubborn and resistant to trying new things (tamasic vāta) and so on. Here is a checklist adapted from Frawley[13] of the three gunas to help you categorize student behaviour.

TABLE 4.9: STUDENT TRAITS OF THE THREE YOGIC GUNAS

	Sattva	**Rajas**	**Tamas**
Self-control	Good	Moderate	Weak
You will notice that some students have good control over their behaviour and reactions. This is partly cultural and partly constitutional. Fiery and airy types often have less self-control, for example, but that doesn't mean the more introverted students are better. It is important to differentiate between self-control and cultural self-expression.			
Speech	Calm and peaceful	Agitated/emotive	Dull
Pay attention to the quality of tone when students speak. You will pick up dullness or agitation in some students, which will give you an indication of what mood they might be in. Your assumption may not be correct, so never assume and never mention what you observe unless a student brings it up first.			
Cleanliness	High	Moderate	Low
Sloppy appearance reflects a certain attitude of mind. However, be careful not to jump to conclusions. There could be very legitimate reasons why students are not clean.			
Attitude in class	Selfless	For personal goals	Lazy
Some students are quite selfish and others more aware of the needs of their colleagues. It is up to you to encourage cooperation and kindness as you run your class.			
Anger	Rarely	Sometimes	Frequently
If you have a pitta aggravated student, they may get angry with you at the drop of a hat. Don't take it personally. It is classic pitta aggravation.			
Fear	Rarely	Sometimes	Frequently
Some students are scared of trying new things. Respect this but be encouraging and try to build up your students' confidence so they feel they can take more risks. It may take quite some time, so be patient.			

13 Frawley, D. (1998). *Āyurveda and the Mind.* Delhi: Motilal Banarsidass. (pp.37–38)

<table>
<tr><td>Desire</td><td>Spiritual</td><td>Mental</td><td>Physical</td></tr>
<tr><td colspan="4">It is up to you to create the general culture of your yoga classes. The goals you set may be a mixture of physical, mental and spiritual, and students will have their own agendas, which may change over time. Students often come to class with physical goals, but as their understanding of the benefits of yoga develop, so do their expectations.</td></tr>
<tr><td>Pride</td><td>Modest</td><td>Vain</td><td>Vain</td></tr>
<tr><td colspan="4">A lot of students need validation from you as their teacher and will develop pride in their practice. Do not discourage this. It may be something they need because they are not getting it elsewhere. One cannot let go of the needs of the ego until it is strong. Vanity is a sign of weakness and is underpinned by insecurity, so it is important to boost confidence.</td></tr>
<tr><td>Depression</td><td>Never</td><td>Sometimes</td><td>Frequently</td></tr>
<tr><td colspan="4">Some students start yoga because they are battling with depression. You may notice or feel their sadness and need to tread carefully around it. Sometimes depressed students prefer to be left alone but most are looking for support. Depression can be more anxious in nature (vāta) or heavy (kapha). You may observe it but must never mention it unless the student chooses to share it with you first. It is not your job to take it on. Make doubly sure you are including these students in every activity.</td></tr>
<tr><td>Love</td><td>Universal</td><td>Personal</td><td>Lacking in love</td></tr>
<tr><td colspan="4">Loving behaviour is a joy to behold in yoga classes and it tends to spread to the other students too. It is a state that comes and goes like any other but should be cherished and cultivated as much as possible.</td></tr>
<tr><td>Violent behaviour</td><td>Never</td><td>Sometimes</td><td>Frequently</td></tr>
<tr><td colspan="4">Luckily, one rarely encounters violent behaviour in yoga classes, but it has been known to happen. You must remain a calm and stable rock in the face of any conflict and not allow your own emotions to enter the fray.</td></tr>
<tr><td>Attachment to money</td><td>Little</td><td>Some</td><td>A lot</td></tr>
<tr><td colspan="4">If a student tries to barter with you, don't assume this is an over-attachment to money. It may be purely cultural. In many countries, bartering is commonplace. Some students, however, will try to avoid payment if they can, and you need to be business-like about this and call it out. You are not running a charity and your time and expertise need to be respected.</td></tr>
<tr><td>Contentment</td><td>Usually</td><td>Partly</td><td>Never</td></tr>
<tr><td colspan="4">Some students are very easy-going and others more demanding. Pitta types tend to be demanding at first until you have proven yourself to them; then they become your most loyal allies. Tamasic students are always unhappy with the class but may keep coming back, regardless. Beyond your usual professional evaluation and self-reflection, don't take this on-board. It is not about you.</td></tr>
<tr><td>Forgiveness</td><td>Forgives easily</td><td>With effort</td><td>Holds long-term grudges</td></tr>
<tr><td colspan="4">We are not perfect, and we all make professional errors when teaching. Most students will forgive these errors, but some won't, and you may find yourself trying to win them over forever more. Don't fall into this cycle.</td></tr>
</table>

<table>
<tr><th></th><th>Sattva</th><th>Rajas</th><th>Tamas</th></tr>
<tr><td>Concentration</td><td>Good</td><td>Moderate</td><td>Poor</td></tr>
<tr><td colspan="4">Some students are really focused on the work and others are constantly distracted, like children. Sometimes a stern word is enough to help these students settle down, especially if they are disrupting the class.</td></tr>
<tr><td>Memory</td><td>Good</td><td>Moderate</td><td>Poor</td></tr>
<tr><td colspan="4">Memory tends to worsen with age, but it can vary according to prakṛti too. Pitta types have good recall wheres in vāta types it is usually very poor. It is just one of those things, but memory can be improved with the right training.</td></tr>
<tr><td>Willpower</td><td>Strong</td><td>Variable</td><td>Weak</td></tr>
<tr><td colspan="4">Pitta types are attracted to strong classes and often have strong willpower, even to their detriment. You will learn to recognize these differences as you get to know your students and understand their needs.</td></tr>
<tr><td>Truthfulness</td><td>Always</td><td>Most of the time</td><td>Rarely</td></tr>
<tr><td colspan="4">Patanjali named satya, or truth, as one of the key Yama in the Yoga Sutras. This is a huge area of spiritual development for all practitioners committed to the yogic path. We are usually unaware of lying to others, because we are lying to ourselves at the same time. It takes a lot of life experience to differentiate between truth and falsehood.</td></tr>
<tr><td>Creativity</td><td>High</td><td>Moderate</td><td>Low</td></tr>
<tr><td colspan="4">Seeing yoga in a fresh way is a sign that creative juices are still flowing. Consider a fresh teaching approach from time to time and see which students react positively.</td></tr>
<tr><td>Meditation</td><td>Daily</td><td>Occasionally</td><td>Never</td></tr>
<tr><td colspan="4">As your students progress and, indeed, as you progress in your practice, meditation will become more and more accessible to you. It is a sign that the mind is settling into its seat (heart) and is less turbulent. It is a genuine sign of spiritual progress, but do not assume that the mind can remain seated in calm. From time to time, emotions will take over and the reactive mind will kick in once more, but it happens less and less frequently.</td></tr>
<tr><td>Service to others</td><td>A lot</td><td>Occasionally</td><td>Never</td></tr>
<tr><td colspan="4">Some students have a strong sense of community and others don't. This, again, is partly cultural and partly to do with temperament. We live in a neo-liberal culture where individuality is considered more important than community spirit. Serving others is a great yoga in itself and many traditions dedicate themselves to it. Consider spending some time in an ashram where you will learn the importance of Karma yoga and seva (service).</td></tr>
<tr><td>Totals</td><td></td><td></td><td></td></tr>
</table>

Chapter 5

VIKṚTI: OUR IMBALANCED SELF

We are all adapting to the demands of life every moment of the day. When agni is strong, those adaptations are barely noticeable. Imbalances rarely last long and we achieve homoeostasis quickly. When we are no longer able to adapt successfully, the body and mind start to display signs of imbalance related to the three doṣas. It is important to remember our wholeness and wellness before the imbalance took hold, otherwise we start to identify with being unwell all the time and it becomes a permanent fixture of our identity, like a lodger taking up permanent residence.

Ageing is a form of adaptation. Our prakṛti fully ripens and we are conscious of all the key facets of our being, but our needs change with age. When we are young, we are generally more physical and sexual, and hungrier for experience; but as we age, we mellow, settle and live more easefully with ourselves. Our prakṛti is still the same, but what we want and what we are able to do may be different.

Most people associate ageing with illness, loss of function and decrepitude, but Āyurveda insists that it doesn't have to be this way. With right living, we should be able to slow down the impact of ageing and limit illness to the period leading up to death itself. I have noticed over the years that when people are completing assessments on prakṛti, they are actually identifying with current personality drives and ailments that arise from their lifestyle rather than enduring character traits. It is quite tricky to differentiate between our true and adapted nature.

When imbalances are corrected, our prakṛti naturally shines through and we begin to smile again because we are coming from an authentic place. We do not need to know why we smile, because smiles arise naturally when we are happy and well. We do, however, need to know what makes us frown so that we know what to avoid or what to be mindful of as we move forwards in life. We are constantly changing, so that sense of naturalness doesn't last forever, unfortunately. Life has more challenges planned for us.

It is certainly true that when we learn to connect with our 'higher self', our 'true nature' naturally arises, and we will live a happier life. Alas, it is not as simple as switching on a light for most of us. We construct false or incomplete versions of ourselves all the time, sometimes without even realizing it. Everyone is prone to self-delusion, even yoga practitioners who adopt 'Buddha-like' personalities and relegate their baser instincts to the unconscious where they eventually wreak havoc.

One of the best ways of helping our students is to share our own journey through life's difficulties as honestly as we can. Āyurveda places great emphasis on self-responsibility, but the issue is complex, and simplistic morality, as often expressed in the old scriptures, is rarely helpful. There are certain key assumptions, which are even perpetuated in yoga and Āyurveda communities, that need to be addressed. One is that there is a perfect state of wellbeing that can be achieved if only we did more of x or y or less of z.

Life is in a constant state of flux and so are we. It is certainly possible to build an inner protective shell through yoga practice and Āyurvedic living, but we are human and should allow ourselves to fully experience the drama of our lives without shame. Life is for living. Don't waste it by sitting on the sidelines and worrying about what other people might think. Trust the journey. Remember that you are not in the driving seat. You cannot change the main milestones of your life, but your reactions to them can change the course of your story.

We mature by making mistakes and, for most of us, the choices we make improve over time because we have adverse reactions that tell us what we don't like. However, it is important to view ourselves as unfinished works. We have an idealized version of ourselves, but prakṛti is in a constant state of flux as it seeks to maintain its integrity in the face of constant challenge. Don't hold on too tightly. Your hand will hurt. Change is the only constant.

> We don't need to know who we are to know who we are not.

> Don't hold on too tightly. Your hand will hurt.

We soon learn that the road to perfect health is full of booby traps that can shake us to the core. We think we know what is working for us, but we are not always correct. Life experiences provide us with clarity about what we want and don't want but they can also give us a false sense of security because we are not always able to differentiate between experiences that are genuinely healthy and those that bring temporary relief but are ultimately harming us.

For example, one glass of wine can calm our nerves, but several glasses will hurt us. In the absence of wisdom from our elders, we rely on our own experience to differentiate between right and wrong actions. We may not fully know everything that can serve us, but Āyurveda tells us in no uncertain terms what is definitely hurting us. There are some universal truths that apply to everyone regardless of their prakṛti.

Change isn't easy. Our lives are propped up by all sorts of distractions and comforts that can obfuscate the core reasons why we are unwell, so it takes courage to stop, clear some space and take a hard look at ourselves. Enthusiasm and willpower can only last so long, and we often end up back where we started. We feel stuck in patterns of behaviour that feel like hamster wheels in our minds: in and out of diets, in and out of relationships, stuck in unwanted jobs, partnerships, eating patterns and so on. It is difficult to consider the possibility of doing things differently, because it would mean changing the way we see ourselves, and change can be terrifying because it feels like a kind of death. Our ego will fight change to the bitter end, which is why we feel that life is initially against us as soon as we try to do things differently.

Our sense of self-identity or ego is essential when we need to protect ourselves, but we end up conserving the familiar even if the habits we have formed are harming us. That protective function gets very nervous when we try to do things differently and needs a lot of reassurance. Change must be gentle and diplomatic. It is a bit like trying to get a child to eat vegetables. You make them into nice shapes, coat them in honey or sneak them into other foods. This is the best way to approach change within us too, but we also need to bear in mind that after a certain age the clock is ticking. Our liver is exhausted; we may be morbidly obese or worse.

The most painful part of the journey is becoming fully conscious of the truth. We lie to ourselves constantly to maintain the status quo and prevent ourselves from hurtling into a state of panic and anxiety. Keeping a diary is a sure-fire way of taking a step back and looking at the things we say to ourselves. It is essential to keep asking the question: Is this really true?

It is essential to keep asking the question: Is this really true?

When I was doing clinical training in India, every couple of weeks a man would be admitted to the hospital with sickness and pain caused by cirrhosis. One might sensibly ask why the man kept on drinking when he knew that the drink was literally killing him. He believed that he would one day find the strength to overcome the habit, that this would be the last time he would be admitted and that things would change for him. By the time we left, he had died.

When we are bombarded with endless adverts for products that make shallow promises, it is easy to think that someone else can take away our suffering for us. However, Āyurveda constantly reminds us that products that bring temporary relief from symptoms we may be experiencing will not ultimately solve our problems. We need to face ourselves, confront our lifestyle habits and get real. In a capitalist world, we must be constantly vigilant of unscrupulous profiteering at our expense. When we have an adverse physical reaction to something, like a certain food, strong wind, extreme cold and heat, an unpleasant person and so on, it is easy to identify a preference and know what we need. However, our ability to recognize what is wrong for us is not always that well developed.

We are all heavily influenced by market forces and cultural norms. It is a fact that all day long we are being manipulated to eat foods that contain sugar, fat and salt. This is an evolutionary response and is very powerful. It takes a great deal of strength and determination to overcome these forces, which is why we must always be kind to ourselves and forgive ourselves when we fall off the wagon.

Action planning

Living with a little danger is part of life. Taking risks invigorates the spirit. However, living with constant danger, especially when it is self-created, is unwise. When embarking on the difficult road to change, there are three points to consider:

1. Most importantly, we have to recognize that there is a problem. If we fool ourselves with delusional statements like 'I can stop this whenever I like' or 'I enjoy it', then we are perpetuating the problem to the point where it really is too late.

2. We have to want to and believe that we can change. Once we identify with a dysfunction by saying things like 'That's just who I am' or 'I'm too old to change', then it becomes a downward spiral that leads to a point of no return.

3. We have to accept that we can't do it alone. If we find ourselves saying things like 'Leave it with me' or 'I created it, so I'll fix it', then our willpower will eventually run out of steam and we will fall back into old habits that have become too powerful to tackle on our own. Don't try and go it alone!

Take a look at the following assessment. It is very similar to the prakṛti constitutional assessment, but this test focuses on our potential imbalances. You can't have eyes everywhere, so I have added an extra column to help you prioritize in order of importance or urgency.

TABLE 5.1: WHAT IS WRONG WITH ME?

	Vāta	Tick	Pitta	Tick	Kapha	Tick	Priority 1–5
Appetite	Too low, rarely hungry		Too high, always hungry for sour and spicy		Too high, always hungry for sweet and salty		
Body weight	Too thin, difficulty putting on weight				Too fat, difficulty losing weight		
Bowel movement	Dry, prone to constipation		Loose, prone to diarrhoea		Bulky, mucus in stool		
Breathing	Shallow, breathless		Chesty and rapid		Obstructed		
Digestive problems	Gas and bloating		Acid indigestion		High mucus and congestion		
Dreams	Fear, flying, being chased		Conflict, anger		Nostalgia, can't get home		
Ears	Ringing, tinnitus		Pain and inflammation		Pus and discharge		
Energy level	Hyperactive, always on the go		Intense, prone to mental exhaustion		Sluggish, difficulty getting motivated		
Eyes	Dry		Red and inflamed		Crusty		
Hair	Dry and brittle, split ends		Bald, grey		Oily, dandruff		
Immunity	Weak, easily gets sick		Food allergies and intolerances (e.g., to red meat, coffee and alcohol)		Respiratory allergies, hay fever, intolerance to gluten and dairy		
Joint health	Cracking and bony		Tender and inflamed		Swollen, numb		

Lips	Dry	Sensitive and inflamed	Swollen, pale
Memory	Very forgetful	Self-centred	Never, ever forgets
Mucus	Too little	Yellow and hot	Copious
Nails	Ridged, dry, brittle	Sensitive, fragile	Thickened, fungal growth
Sex drive	High libido but passes quickly	Angry when unsatisfying	Low libido, can't initiate
Skin	Dark hue, dry, rough	Red and oily, spots, rashes, eczema, psoriasis	White, pallid
Sleep	Difficulty going to sleep, disturbed 2–6am	Disturbed 12–2am	Difficulty waking up or getting up
Spine	Lower back pain	Pain in mid-back or shoulder blades	Bone spurs, abnormal growth
Stress response	Freeze with fear or run away	Angry and confrontational	Indifferent, uncaring, unresponsive
Thirst	Forget to drink water	Always thirsty for cold drinks	Drink out of habit rather than thirst
Tongue	Dry, no coat	Bright red and wet, dirty yellow coat	Pale and swollen, thick white coat
Urine	Scanty	Burning and yellow	Copious, mucus, white and frothy
Voice	Breathy, dry tone, stuttering or stammering	Sharp, bossy and uncaring	Slow to express, depressing, monotonous

— Chapter 6 —

AGNI AND ĀMA

Agni (fire) is a useful metaphor adopted by Āyurveda which encapsulates a whole number of processes that support life. It is a very old concept that originated in the *Rig Veda*, about 5000 years ago. It was a time when agni was worshipped as a deity (Agni Deva) but in the modern Āyurvedic paradigm, it is still a useful symbol, as we will see.

On a macrocosmic level, agni represents solar energy. In many respects, we are children of the sun. We are sustained by its life-giving light and the food that it produces. We are dependent on the sun in every way, and the life that we lead is like a minute splinter that burns brightly for a time and then fades.

This is why the concept of agni is so important. In many Āyurvedic books it is loosely interpreted as digestive fire, but it is much more than that. It represents the health of our entire metabolism. The strength of our agni is always the first consideration in any health condition. Low agni could be the cause or the outcome of disease. It is incumbent on all of us to take care of our agni, especially as we age, because it naturally diminishes with time.

Agni and yoga

Agni is central to all classical yoga practices and is a central goal in all yoga practices of the *HYP*. When teaching yoga from an Āyurvedic perspective, working with agni should be up there in the top three themes.

Most people think that agni is all about digestion and, in one sense, this is true. There are many expressions of agni but the most important is jaṭhara agni, which is the fire that drives the digestive processes. Jaṭhara means 'abdomen', so jaṭhara agni refers to all the digestive functions that are fulfilled by the abdominal viscera. This includes the stomach, pancreas, small and large intestines and, most importantly, the liver.

The *Caraka Saṃhitā* mentions over 40 specialized agnis, but jaṭhara agni is the most important because it is located at the main interface between the outside world and our body. Whatever gets processed by jaṭhara agni eventually becomes us. The quality of what we eat as well as the quality of our cooking equipment will ultimately be reflected in the quality of our tissues. Poor-quality food inevitably leads to the formation of āma, a morbid toxic material that clogs the channels and produces poor-quality dhātus or tissues. Low agni can impair the following functions, as laid out by Vasant Lad in the first volume of his book *Textbook of Āyurveda:*[1]

- **Pakti:** This word means 'digestion' but also 'ripening', so it refers to the proper digestion of food but also the assimilation of other types of food that stimulate our senses, including what we take in as sight, sound, smell, touch and taste. Ripening is important and refers to the proper formation of the dhātus or tissues that make up the body. Unripe tissues have weak immunity and are vulnerable to assault and accumulation of toxins. Finally, pakti also refers to our mind's ability to assimilate knowledge and information. A cloudy and muddled mind is a sign of low agni.

- **Darśana:** Literally means 'viewing' or 'seeing'. It can simply refer to visual perception but also touches on the idea of mental clarity and understanding. Clouded perception is one sign of low agni.

- **Mātrosna:** 'Matra', meaning 'measurement', is coupled with the word 'uṣṇa', which means 'hot', so mātrosna means 'right amount of heat or body temperature'. Low agni can cause a drop in body temperature.

1 Lad, V. (2002). *Textbook of Āyurveda*, Volume 1. Albuquerque, NM: The Ayurvedic Press. (p.86)

- **Prakṛti varna:** Varna means 'colour' or 'outward appearance'. We all have a unique complexion and when agni is strong, we have good colour and lustre.
- **Śauryam:** This word is used in the *Bhagavad Gita*[2] and refers to the courage and valour needed to fight a war. When we have low agni, we lose the will to fight for what we want.
- **Harṣā:** Means 'happiness' or 'delight', which is a natural state we observe in children but lose over time as agni diminishes.
- **Prasāda:** Literally means 'gracious gift',[3] and is akin to the abundant mindset of the gods. We feel abundant and generous with ourselves and others when we are well.
- **Rāga:** Means 'passion or zest for life'.
- **Dhātu poṣaṇam:** The proper formation of bodily tissues.
- **Ojaskara:** The proper formation of ojas, the essence of kapha doṣa. Controls all immunity functions.
- **Tejaskara:** The proper formation of tejas, the essence of pitta doṣa. Controls all transformative functions and the quality of radiance.
- **Prāṇa kara:** The proper formation of prāṇa, the essence of vāta doṣa. Controls vital energy and all movement and coordination of bodily functions.
- **Medhākara:** The proper formation of general intelligence (IQ).
- **Buddhi:** The wisdom mind. When the mind is less clouded, we have greater access to its broader functions, including intuition and intellect, which are functions of buddhi.
- **Dhairyam:** Means 'patience' or 'forbearance'. When agni is strong, we are less impulsive and have much greater capacity for endurance.

---

2 *Bhagavad Gita*, Verse 43, Chapter 18. Accessed on 31/3/21 https://gitajourney.com//?s=verse+43&search=Go.

3 Wisdom Library (2021) Prasada. Accessed on 18/2/2021 https://www.wisdomlib.org/definition/prasada.

- **Dīrgha:** Literally means 'for a long time' and refers to our lifespan. Maintaining strong agni is the key to longevity in Āyurveda.
- **Prabhā:** Means 'light', 'glow, or 'shine' and refers to the lustre of our skin.
- **Bala:** Means 'strength' and normally refers to the robustness of our body.
- **Constitutional strength:** Some people have naturally strong constitutions. We all know who they are because they rarely get sick despite their lifestyle. Most of us are not that lucky and the older we get, the harder we need to work to maintain our strength and immunity.

Types of agni imbalance

There are many considerations when assessing the strength of our agni. A sluggish liver is a major contributor to all agni imbalances and deserves some attention on its own. The first thing to assess is the bowel movement because it reflects the health of jaṭhara agni, the digestive fire. If jaṭhara agni is low, this has a knock-on effect all the way down to tissue formation and, ultimately, mental health. Here are the four tendencies of jaṭhara agni:

- **Samāgni (balanced agni):** Your bowel movement is normal. It moves at least once a day, comes out smoothly and appears like a ripe banana in consistency (not colour!). The colour should be brown, but its shade will depend on what you eat.
- **Viṣamāgni (irregular agni):** Commonly associated with vāta aggravation. There is no consistency. Sometimes it is dry and hard, sometimes runny, and it can move at any time of the day or not at all.
- **Tīkṣṇāgni (sharp agni):** Commonly associated with pitta aggravation. The bowel is loose and runny, often hot with burning sensations. There may be bits of undigested food. Can move several times day.

- **Mandāgni (slow agni):** Bowel movement is slow, bulky and heavy. There may be mucus, which will make it stick to the edge of the pan.

What a Yoga teacher needs to know about agni

Now that you have a sense of what agni is and how to recognize low agni, there are a few things you can offer your students without overstepping your professional boundaries. An Āyurvedic practitioner trains for a long time to understand the subtleties of therapeutic intervention. You are not trying to do that. You are simply empowering your students with a basic understanding of the concept of agni and giving them some ideas about what they can do for themselves. For anything beyond this, you should refer your student to a practitioner.

Environment

It is very difficult to maintain optimal agni in the current environment. When the air, water and food all have contaminants, the body needs to work very hard to sustain wellness. Experts say that the liver has to process a multitude of toxins a day, so inevitably, it is an uphill struggle. We need to be mindful of what we can control and make every effort to reduce the toxic load on the body by eating well, drinking pure water, keeping away from electromagnetic pollutants and taking time to get out of the city.

Diet

Good-quality food cannot fully compensate for constitutionally low agni but it can go a long way towards sustaining wellness. Digestive fire can be vastly improved with the right herbs and foods.

Here are some key agni kindling foods:

- Fermented foods like kefir, kombucha and sauerkraut
- Fresh fruit and vegetables

- Ghee
- Pungent, spicy foods like onions and mustard
- Fresh sour foods like berries, lemon and lime.

Herbs that kindle agni

To help you choose the most useful herbs, it is important to have a sense of what kind of agni you have. Ideally, we are all aiming for balanced agni, but if we have slow agni, we will not be using the same herbs as if we have sharp agni. In fact, the wrong herbs can make a problem worse.

Here are two key herbs you should definitely use:

- **Ginger:** Known as the 'universal medicine'. Ginger is sweet and pungent in taste with a hot potency. The powder is hotter than the root because it is drier. It is a very ubiquitous herb that is useful for clearing cold and improving circulation and is an excellent anti-inflammatory, particularly in arthritic conditions. It is a well-known remedy for nausea.
- **Black pepper:** Pungent and bitter in taste with a hot potency. An excellent āma pāchana or toxin cooker. Its strong pungent action helps clear the head of congestion but also has the power to kill pathogens and clear channels.

The following herbs are also good agni dīpanas (agni kindlers).

- Cinnamon
- Cardamon
- Cumin
- Coriander
- Cloves
- Fennel
- Turmeric
- Rock salt
- Aloe vera
- Lemon
- Lime
- Mint

Emotional health

Agni is strongly affected by negative emotions. If you are experiencing high levels of stress, you will notice that your agni diminishes and this will eventually impact on your bowel movements. If you are going through a difficult and stressful period, try to compensate by taking more agni-kindling herbs and eating well.

Daily routines

Proper daily routines have a huge impact on the health of your agni:

- **Poor sleep:** This can seriously impair agni if it goes on for too long. Take steps to improve your sleep as much as possible using herbs, foods and adequate exercise.
- **Timely meals:** Eating at irregular times can impact your agni. Try to eat at similar times every day. It is scientifically proven that the later in the day you consume food, the slower the calories burn off. If you are trying to lose weight, take this point seriously and follow the golden rule:

  Breakfast like a princess

  Lunch like a queen

  Dinner like a pauper
- **Exercise:** Try to raise your heart rate for at least 20 minutes three times a week. Exercise is one of the easiest and most important ways of strengthening your agni. You were designed to move, so your body needs it. Children never stop moving because it is natural for them to do so. We need to rekindle our childlike spirit and learn to play with movement rather than seek out enjoyment on a computer screen.

How strong is your agni?

Agni impacts every aspect of our health, so we can safely assume that any imbalance will be related to it in some way. However, when we want to assess the state of our agni in isolation, we can contextualize the various aspects in order to make sense of them. Here is a short test.

TABLE 6.1: HOW STRONG IS YOUR AGNI?

Enquiry	Samāgni (normal)	Tick	Viṣamāgni (irregular)	Tick	Tīkṣṇāgni (sharp)	Tick	Mandāgni (slow)	Tick	Priority level 1–5
Bowel movement	Smooth, regular		Hard, irregular		Hot, runny		Sticky, solid		
Digestive power (pakti)	Good appetite		Irregular appetite		Voracious appetite		Low appetite		
Perception (darśana)	Good awareness		Unable to concentrate for long		Intense concentration		Dull, unmotivated		
Immunity (ojas kara)	Able to recover normally		Delicate health, easily sick		Prone to inflammation, otherwise strong		Prone to congestive disorders, long time to recover		
Senses (indriya pakti)	All senses work normally		Hearing sensitive		Sensitive vision		Acute sense of smell		
Quality of tissues (dhātu poṣaṇam)	Normal body development		Difficulty putting on weight, weak bones and joints		Blood and skin disorders, inflammatory conditions		Excess fat		
Body temperature (mātrosna)	Normal		Cold hands and feet		Burning sensations, feel hot all the time		Low circulation, feel cold		
Complexion (prakṛti varna)	Normal		Dry, sallow		Red, oily		White		
Radiance (tejas kara)	Bright		Dull		Red		Poor		
Courage (śauryam)	Willing to take calculated risks		Reticent and fearful		Angry and reactive, unwise risks.		Will avoid anything risky		

Enquiry	Samāgni (normal)	Tick	Viṣamāgni (irregular)	Tick	Tīkṣṇāgni (sharp)	Tick	Mandāgni (slow)	Tick	Priority level 1–5
Intelligence (medhākara)	Good balance between emotion and intellect		Unsettled mind, unable to apply intelligence for long		Overly sharp, intolerant and judgemental		Dull mind, slow at learning and understanding		
Wisdom. clarity of mind (buddhi)	Able to assess situations and see all sides		Emotionally over-whelmed easily and unable to see the big picture		Obsessed with one point of view only		Unmotivated, dull, indifferent		
Happiness	Good balance		Extremely happy or sad		Happy only when engaged in something intense		Narrow field of experience, prone to depression		
Abundance	Good balance		Always struggling to make ends meet		Never enough		Hoarding impulse		
Passion for life (rāga)	Want to engage		Short lived		Overly intense		Indifferent		
Energy levels	Good		Short bursts		Extremes followed by complete exhaustion		Low		
Patience (dhairyam)	Good		Low		Low		Indifferent about the outcome		
Longevity (dīrgha)	Good		Low		Low		Low		
Skin lustre (prabhā)	Good		Darkish		Reddish		Whitish		
Strength (bala)	Good		Weak		Overuse		Underuse		

— Chapter 7 —

ĀYURVEDA IN ĀSANA TEACHING

We have reached a point where we can now revisit the familiar with an Āyurvedic lens. Āsana means 'posture'. It is mentioned in a variety of important texts including Patanjali's *Yoga Sutras* and, of course, the *HYP*. The goal of āsana practice can be set within a broader yogic paradigm as well as a more specific Āyurvedic one. Āsana may be considered as one of the preparatory practices for deeper meditative work or it can be an integral part of healthy living with Āyurvedic principles.

The practice and benefits of āsana practice may be considered from the point of view of the panchakoshas or five sheaths of the body as mentioned in the *Taittirīyopaniṣad*.[1]

Annamayakośa (food sheath – physical body)

When we are communicating the benefits of āsana to our students, it is important to start with what is immediately known and experienced by all, especially beginners. We experience āsana through the physical body and can explain the benefits of movement and posture purely in these terms.

The key physical goals of āsana practice would be to seek postural

1 Satyananda Saraswati, Swami (2004). *Nine Principal Upaniṣads*. Bihar: Yoga Publications Trust. (pp.232–237)

integrity through the exploration of right relationship between our body and the ground. Postural imbalances caused by lifestyle habits, such as long sitting or standing or using one side of the body excessively, lead to physical imbalances that bring about pain and discomfort. Regular āsana practice can be a powerful and effective method of helping the body to rediscover its own postural integrity.

> The key physical goals of āsana practice would be to seek postural integrity.

Postural integrity involves the proper relationship between all the moving parts, especially the connective tissue or fascia that binds us together and gives us a sense of ourselves as a unified physical being rather than the individual functioning parts therein. It is more useful to view our bodies in this way than try to analyse the functions of individual working parts such as muscles, joints and bones. We are more like balloons than robots in the sense that we cannot isolate a localized event without taking the rest of the body into account. For example, if we pull a muscle in our leg, this apparent localized event will impact the rest of our body. When we press one side of an inflated balloon, the rest of the balloon stretches to compensate.

Prāṇamayakośa (pranic sheath – vital body)

When we assess our experience of āsana practice from a subtle or energetic perspective, we notice that with regular practice, we not only begin to feel freer in our bodies, but also have more energy and endurance. Āyurveda explains this by presenting us with the prāṇic body. According to Āyurveda, our physical body would be inanimate without the presence of prāṇa, much like a car without an electrical system. Our aliveness depends on our body's ability to generate energy. Every cell actually has its own independent capacity to generate energy and this ultimately extends to our whole being.

Prāṇa means 'that which animates' so, in that sense, it is the driving force behind everything. The word 'prāṇa' can mean slightly different things according to the context in which it is written. It can represent the whole cosmos as an energy field, or it can represent the functioning of our mind and body.

From an Āyurvedic perspective, prāṇa and vāta are actually one. Prāṇa is said to be the essence of vāta, but vāta has no substance per se, so they are one and the same in this sense. Vāta relates to specific functions and dysfunctions of prāṇa.

In the previous chapters we learned that vāta represents the moving principle, so it controls the movement of everything that comes into the body, moves around the body and leaves the body.

When we are practising āsana, we are enabling the free and harmonious flow of vāta or prāṇa from the core of the body right through to our very extremes. When vāta is impaired, we experience pain, blockage and a lack of mobility. Āsana can really help to free up the flow of prāṇa so that we experience the benefits not only physically but also in our energy field.

When we are working with āsana, we can impact on our prāṇic body in the following ways:

- Āsana groups can impact our prāṇic body differently. For example, back bends can make us feel more vital, and forward bends can make us feel more relaxed.
- Our experience of an āsana itself can vary depending on how we use the breath. Focusing more on exhalations, for example, can help us maintain calm, whereas the inhalation can enliven us.
- By liberating prāṇic blockages around the marma zones, our prāṇic body can flourish and we are motivated to embrace life with more enthusiasm.

By liberating prāṇic blockages around the marma zones, our prāṇic body can flourish and we are motivated to embrace life with more enthusiasm.

Manomayakośa (mental sheath – field of thought and emotion)

Āsana can be practised as a form of meditation. By observing the quality of our thoughts during practice, we become aware of the impact of the mental gunas or qualities on our practice.

- **Rajas:** This represents the dynamic force that can unsettle the mind and prevent us from being present in the practice.
- **Tamas:** This represents a dull state of mind that can also prevent us from being present because we feel deadened and unmotivated.

Both gunas need to be tempered with sattva, which represents clarity, detachment and equanimity. A high level of sattva can prevent excessive rajas or tamas from sabotaging the work. If we pay attention to how we feel during the practice, we will notice that our feelings are affecting the way we think, and this can affect the quality of our entire practice.

As soon as we lose that control over our minds, it is best to come out of the posture, take a break and do it again. Persistence slowly builds stamina, and we find that we are also more able to cope with life's challenges in general. (See Table 4.9.)

Vijñānamayakośa (wisdom sheath – field of higher understanding)

Vijnana means 'higher understanding'[2] and represents the buddhi or wisdom mind. It is believed that our buddhi acts as a kind of intermediary between our manas (cognitive or lower mind) and our soul or Ātman. Our buddhi informs us through our intuition of what is right or wrong for us, whether we are on the right track, so to speak. The more we practise yoga, the better our relationship with buddhi becomes. We learn to trust our intuition more and more and notice that our choices pave a better way.

---

2 Feuerstein, G. (1990). *Encyclopaedic Dictionary of Yoga*. London: Unwin Health. (p.392)

Ānandamayakośa (bliss sheath – field of complete absorption)

We get glimmers of our bliss sheath when we have peak experiences. Some say we are made of the stuff of god and god is love, so in essence we are bodies of bliss. Bliss usually arises momentarily and passes, but the more we align ourselves with our Prakṛti, the more we are likely to attract experiences that bring us joy and bliss because our activities mirror our true nature.

A life well lived is a life of deep satisfaction and purpose. For some of us, that purpose remains obscured till later in life; for others, it is there from the beginning. Children are naturally drawn to experiences that make them happy, until adults discourage them and sometimes steer them in another direction. It can take a long time to reconnect with that childhood instinct and live in peace with ourselves. The bliss sheath is a thin veil that separates us from oneness, the ultimate loss of separateness.

One of the reasons students come back to āsana practice is because it gives them heightened experiences. When prāṇa is released from a shackled state caused by poor posture or lack of movement, the body and mind often experience a flush of bliss as a reward for right action. This rush of endorphins doesn't always happen immediately. There can be a lot of resistance at first and that blissful feeling that comes from practice grows gradually over a longer period of time. It is a sign that we have stirred something deep and true because our body and mind sing our praises. It is also common for this so-called 'blissed out' feeling to subside. The body reaches a new equilibrium and no longer rewards us, because we have created a new normal.

Many students lose motivation after this occurs and allow themselves to get blocked up again so that they can be rewarded all over again. At the other end of the spectrum, students will push themselves harder and harder in the quest for new highs and end up hurting themselves.

Āsana is designed to bring us into balance. Once this is achieved, we should move on to more subtle practices like prāṇāyāma and meditation, as recommended by the *HYP*. In classical yoga, āsana was never meant to be a complete practice in and of itself.

How to work in āsana with an Āyurvedic perspective

There are two fundamental ways of viewing āsana practice:

- Shape
- Direction

Shape

An āsana is a dynamic shape one creates with the body. This shape is dynamic because the body is actively engaged with it. There is no stillness, no stasis. Every inch of the body is consciously engaged. Every part has its role to play. Some parts are more important than others, but there are no redundant parts. Āsana is like matter itself. When you look closely enough, all parts of the body are fully alive.

From a distance, the body may look static but up close, it isn't. This contradiction is important. The reason why the body looks static from a distance is because the movement is subtle. Āsana practice should progress in a gentle way, especially later on when the student has learned to become more kinaesthetically aware.

Every shape impacts the body on different levels. A shape can emulate sacred geometry like circles, spirals, triangles and squares. Each of these shapes is used by Prakṛti to represent different ideas and frequencies in nature. For example, traditionally, triangles were considered to be harmonious and squares more dynamic and tension generating. Every āsana is a combination of different shapes interacting with each other. Back bends, for example, always have a circular quality as the spine hyperextends, and poses where arms and legs are abducted can create different angles in relation to the midline. Vīrabhadrāsana 2 (Warrior 2) creates more squares, for example, and Trikoṇāsana (Triangle pose) obviously creates more triangles.

Direction

Skilful āsana practice comes with an understanding of which way things are going. Directions of movement are layered.

The first consideration is in knowing what to give to the ground and what to move away from the ground. What goes up and what comes down. Using the breath plays an intimate part in us. We generally use the inhalation to move away from the ground and the exhalation to surrender to the ground.

Beyond that, direction is created by knowing about the key articulations we need to work within a posture. It is important to point out that there is no one way of doing any posture. There is only your way and my way or our teacher's way. There are many versions of Trikoṇāsana (Triangle pose) for example, and none of them are wrong; they are just different. It is important to know what you want your students to experience when practising a posture, because every variation creates a slightly different shape. Every technique highlights a slightly different focus.

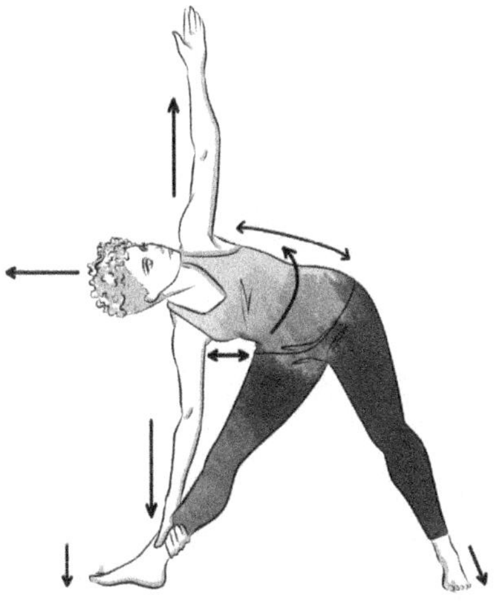

Figure 7.1: Directions of Trikoṇāsana (Triangle Pose)

Let's take a closer look at Trikoṇāsana (Triangle pose). In Iyengar's version of Trikoṇāsana (Triangle pose), the arms are externally rotated at the shoulder joints, but the lower arm is internally rotated at the elbow joint to make a spiral. Try that now, so you know what I mean. We look at the visual shape of Trikoṇāsana (Triangle pose) and that gives us one sense. Then we study more closely the ways in which the overall shape is opening up the body. Where is the space being created as the āsana moves towards its full expression?

> Where is the space being created as the āsana moves towards its full expression?

Recognizing this is an important step in becoming more conscious. We want to make all our sheaths conscious, not just the ones we prefer. Some practitioners are less interested in the body and naturally gravitate toward experiences in the subtle sheaths. If you neglect the practices of a particular sheath, you could be paving the way for an imbalance later on.

Practise with awareness

There is nothing, and I mean *nothing*, more important in yoga practice than practising with awareness. Before you can even start to practise yoga with an Āyurvedic approach, you need to know yourself. Who is it that is practising?

There is a contradiction in this guideline because when we start practising yoga, we are largely ignorant of who we are. Rare is the student who is kinaesthetically aware from the start. In this case, a student should go to classes and practise a set sequence at home. This book is not for them, it is for you. You are a yoga teacher, presumably at a point in your practice where you are reasonably self-aware and have attained a certain degree of competence in your practice.

> There is nothing, and I mean *nothing*, more important in yoga practice than practising with awareness.

The overall development and expansion of an āsana leads to greater spaciousness within the joints and ultimately all the tissues of the body, but this is impossible without a conscious awareness of the former.

Some students find it easier to work backwards. In other words, they see the shape you are creating, try to copy it and expect their bodies to work out how to do so in an intuitive way. This certainly works for those who have hidden kinaesthetic intelligence, but for most people more explicit guidance is much more helpful.

Consciously engaging in the mechanics of āsana practice is an ideal way of keeping the mind focused. It is a concrete task that the mind can easily grasp and work on. The mind needs this, and the body needs it too.

If we are not conscious of what we are doing with our bodies, āsana practice can become unsafe because we do not pick up red lights in time. We might end up over-compressing joints, holding the body in misalignment or forcing the body into a position that it is not ready for. We have to be conscious and act wisely, otherwise āsana can end up being one of the many things we do in life with Prajñāparādha – crime against wisdom.

Āsana practice is cultivating the right balance between:

- When to push and when to allow
- When to give and when to take
- When to move and when to be still
- When to hold firm and when to let go.

Āsana and the doṣas

Vāta doṣa

We know so far that vāta controls all movement and communication of the body. If vāta controls movement, then it will inevitably play a major part in āsana practice. We are also reminded of the following:

- The primary seat of vāta is in the colon.
- Vāta controls the hours of 2am–6am and 2pm–6pm.
- The secondary seats of vāta are the organs in the same lower band in which the kidneys lie, including the kidneys, lower back and bladder. It also settles in our bones, joints and skin.
- A vāta-aggravated person is likely to experience viṣamāgni, which means 'irregular agni', where the bowel moves at irregular times and constantly changes between hard and soft stools.

The qualities or gunas of vāta are:

- Dry
- Light
- Cold
- Rough
- Subtle
- Mobile
- Clear

We can take these qualities to a deeper level of causation. Gunas can be aggravated due to endogenous factors (what's happening within us) but also due to exogenous factors (environmental).

Internal causes usually come about as a result of how we live. All endogenous causes can be considered from three points of view:

- **Atiyoga:** Overuse of our body and senses.
- **Ayoga:** Underuse of our body and senses.
- **Mithyā yoga:** Misuse of our body and senses.

Inappropriate practice can contribute to vāta imbalances. The key imbalances of vāta are:

- Blocked vāta (sanga)
- Excessive flow of vāta (atipravṛtti)
- Misdirected flow of vāta (vimārga gamanam).

This approach also applies to the way we practise āsana itself. We practise postures that come more easily and as few of those postures that are uncomfortable or difficult as we can get away with. This includes the way we move our body in the āsana itself.

When one part of us won't move, we compensate by moving another part more than we should and potentially injure ourselves. A good example is when we do back bends. Most of us have stiff midbacks and often compensate by bending into our lower backs and necks more than we should. Sustained compression can cause imbalance, leading to injury. This is overuse of the lower back (atiyoga) and underuse of the midback (ayoga) caused by a misuse (mithyā yoga) of the intellect.

We may start off by pleading ignorance. After all, kinaesthetic awareness doesn't come that easily to many. It certainly didn't for me.

I learned the hard way: injury after injury. But I learned in the end. No shortcuts.

To have an understanding of what might happen when vāta is blocked, overactive or misdirected, we need to remind ourselves of the five winds or sub-doṣas of vāta.

- **Apāna:** Seated in the colon and moves downwards and outwards.
- **Udāna:** Seated in the throat and moves upwards and outwards.
- **Prāṇa:** Seated in the head and chest and moves inwards and downwards.
- **Samāna:** Seated in the digestive tract and moves side to side and centripetally towards the navel.
- **Vyāna:** Seated in the heart and moves outwards towards the extremities.

When we are considering the shape and direction of an āsana, we are working to harmonize the five vayus. If one of the vayus is sluggish or blocked, we are using āsana to free it so that it can fulfil its functions properly. For example, apāna vayu controls all downward functions like bowel movements and menstruation. If apāna vayu is blocked or impaired in some way, we may experience constipation, and tightness and stiffness in the hips, lower back and legs. Āsana, along with other Āyurvedic techniques, can help to correct that.

When we are considering the direction of a posture, it is worth bearing this in mind. That way we can prioritize āsana in order of importance from the point of view of which functions we need to correct.

- **Vyāna vayu:** Dynamic standing poses like Vīrabhadrāsana 1 (Warrior 1), Vīrabhadrāsana 2 (Warrior 2) and Trikoṇāsana (Triangle pose) are excellent for improving circulation towards the extremities.
- **Samāna vayu:** Twists and forward bends are good at squeezing and toning the abdomen to help harmonize the flow of samāna vayu.
- **Apāna vayu:** Hip-opening poses (from the front) like Trikoṇāsana,

Vīrabhadrāsana 2 (Warrior 2) and Utthita Pārśvakoṇāsana (Extended Side Angle pose) are good for clearing excess vāta or releasing blocked vāta from its primary seat.

- **Udāna vayu:** Dynamic poses like Utkaṭāsana (Powerful pose), Vīrabhadrāsana 1 (Warrior 1) and Vīrabhadrāsana 3 (Warrior 3) are good for raising energy and galvanizing udāna vayu.
- **Prāṇa vayu:** Back bends and standing poses help to create more space and freedom in the ribcage and create a good foundation for prāṇāyāma practice.

BLOCKED VĀTA

When vāta is blocked, we experience pain in that part of the body, but vāta cannot be unblocked by force. What is blocking vāta? The Āyurvedic texts say that kapha and pitta can block vāta and it can even block itself. What does that mean? When the doṣas have become dysfunctional because of imbalanced agni, the tissues they are associated with start to form in excess or end up depleted. Kapha imbalance can lead to excess fat, for example. Moreover, tissues are unable to fend off toxins, which could also end up blocking the channels. Even toxins will have a resonance with the doṣas. Most toxins of chemical nature, for example, cause inflammation, which aggravates pitta doṣa initially but eventually lead to tridoshic imbalances whereby acids (pitta), mucus (kapha) and various nefarious gases (vāta) build up in the body. If kapha is blocking vāta, the tissues and substances associated with vāta are in excess.

Excess fat is a sign that kapha is aggravated and could be blocking vāta. Fatty plaque inside our arteries could eventually lead to heart disease.

Excess mucus can clog our lungs and sinuses and we would find it difficult to breathe. Kapha uses mucus as a key lubricant, but in excess it will cause swelling and obstruction.

Injury can block vāta because it causes inflammation and swelling. The pain forces us to rest and await recovery. We can take agents that will speed up the reduction of inflammation, such as anti-inflammatory herbs, food and drugs, but ultimately vāta needs to be able to move freely again. Vāta needs to be able to move through an injury to bring healing nutrients and prāṇa to the zone, which is why it is important not to allow too much protective resistance to build up. Trying to move an area of your back or even a broken leg or arm once the tissue has hardened can be extremely painful and we are inclined to want to give up, so it is important to understand this point.

EXCESSIVE VĀTA

When vāta is overactive, it usually means that the mobile quality of vāta is out of balance: you simply cannot stop moving either physically or mentally. When I was younger, I was addicted to sport and exercise. Obviously, wanting to be active is not a bad thing unless it is hurting you; I didn't realize that it was. I was overdoing it because I was unable to rest. I was compensating for all sorts of emotional problems with more and more exercise and this eventually led to my first back injury. More is not always better. It is important to cultivate an understanding of one's stress responses, which are learned early in life and maintain a memory of the negative impact of wrong action. I lacked kinaesthetic intelligence and was unable to differentiate between addictive behaviour and genuine need. I was displacing emotional imbalances and trying to solve them by wearing myself out physically. Unfortunately, I not only wore myself out but wore myself down too.

MISDIRECTED VĀTA

We know that vāta moves in five principal directions and each direction controls a certain number of associated functions. When vāta is blocked, like the wind, it not only brings pain, but can also start to move in a direction it is not meant to, thus creating problems elsewhere in the body.

A good example of this is when we have constipation. Apāna vayu, the downward flow of vāta, may be blocked for any number of reasons, but the consequence isn't just that we are holding a lot of poo. The rebound effect of apāna vayu can cause chest pain, stomach upset and headaches. I have seen many examples of this in my clinic over the years where what appears to be a problem in the head actually originates in the colon.

Another example of misdirected vāta is 'shifting pain'. Sometimes, clients complain of pain that shifts around the body. First it is on one part of the back, then another, then one side of the body, then the other, and so on. The origin of this can also be attributed to misdirected vāta. It may be because apāna vayu is blocked in the colon, or there may be another vayu involved. Another common imbalance is in samāna vayu in the digestive tract. When we have digestive problems that lead to inflammation in the gut lining, damage, leaky gut or stagnation caused by exercise too close to mealtimes, this can easily cause misdirected vāta. Samāna is prevented from doing its job and this leads to all sorts of potential misfires around the body. Āyurveda is very clear about the importance of ritualizing eating and this is one of the most important reasons for doing so.

By practising āsana regularly and mindfully, it is possible to maintain a good balance between the five vayus as long as they are not being blocked by an excess of pitta or kapha doṣa.

VĀTA AND ĀSANA PRACTICE

From an Āyurvedic perspective, identifying the nature and causes of vāta imbalance will be the main key that unlocks our health. If we do not address vāta blockage caused by lifestyle choices that raise pitta and kapha doṣa, it will be difficult to bring vāta into balance and keep it in balance for long.

VĀTA AND SPATIAL AWARENESS

Right relationship of matter in space goes to the heart of what vāta is all about. Vāta represents the animating force. It drives all movement of substance and intelligence. Right communication and collaboration between cells is vāta's job. If cells are unable to coordinate themselves, then all manner of developmental issues can occur. I recently watched a TV programme about a boy in Uganda who was born with a huge tumour on his face that just got bigger and bigger and ended up being as heavy as the head itself. This abnormal growth from an Āyurvedic perspective is a loss of intelligence causing kapha, the growth principle, to become dysfunctional. Right relationship enables everything in our body to be in its place and work in harmony with everything else.

POSTURAL MISALIGNMENTS

When we are young, we are usually very active. We do not think twice about running, jumping and playing. But as we settle into an adult way of life, many of us get into habitual positions for hours on end and this creates postural imbalances. If we do not address these imbalances, the older we get, the harder it is to redress the problems because our tissues normalize the imbalance.

As I sit at my desk writing this book, I am aware that tension is building up in my upper trapezius. My head is crooked forwards, forcing my neck muscles to work harder to support the head. My neck muscles virtually turn into straps to compensate for the misalignment. If I didn't do yoga every day, this would become chronic and I would have a lot of pain to manage.

> Where there is pain, there is vāta.

Yoga helps to correct misalignments caused mainly by lifestyle so that vāta can regain its integrity and help sustain right relationship with the ground. I could write a whole book on this subject alone, but there are already books dedicated to this. We understand a huge amount about pain and movement these days and much of this knowledge is already helping us become better yoga teachers.

THE GUNAS OF VĀTA

Next, we should consider the key gunas that cause us aggravation. We are all different, so not every guna related to vāta is prone to imbalances. For example, dry or raw food may have little impact on vāta if our digestion is strong, but excessive exercise might. When we first adopt an Āyurvedic approach, we take a broad-sweep approach and try to identify the aggravating factors over time.

The general approach to vāta pacifying through āsana should be as follows. Practice should:

- **Be consistent:** Too much stopping and starting will aggravate the irregular or erratic nature of vāta.
- **Be moderate:** Extreme effort or exhaustion will only aggravate vāta more.
- **Be gentle:** Undue stress and force in āsana can cause more injury.
- **Be rhythmic and repetitive:** Vāta needs routine; practising the same sequence mindfully every day can prevent vāta retaliation.
- **Be slow and dynamic leading to stable and still:** Vāta needs to move; too much stillness, especially at the start of the practice will not relieve vāta blockage; movement must be mindful and deliberate.
- **Include joint mobilisation:** As a major part of āsana practice to ensure the proper flow of prāṇa through the marma zones.
- **Emphasize the hip and pelvic region:** This is where vāta is primarily seated.
- **Emphasize spine mobility:** To improve overall posture and whole-body integrity.

SIGNS OF IMPROPER PRACTICE

- **Pain:** You experience more pain not less. Sometimes skilled adjustments by trained practitioners such as osteopaths can cause more pain initially but usually lead to great relief once vāta has settled. This kind of approach should be avoided unless you are an extremely experienced practitioner and know how to manipulate your own body.
- **Stiffness:** If you notice that practice is making you stiffer rather than more supple, you are practising too strongly. It is very likely that you have āma or toxicity that is causing stiffness, so you need to do more than just āsana to overcome it. Seek the advice of an

experienced practitioner, who may put you on a broader regimen that includes diet, herbs and lifestyle changes.

- **Fear and anxiety:** If you notice yourself getting more and more ungrounded, vāta is going up not down. Something is wrong. You are either practising too strongly or the causative factors are too strong for you to manage on your own with yoga. You need to adopt a broader range of vāta-pacifying strategies, including relaxation, breathing and possibly oleation.
- **Insomnia:** This became an issue for me when I first started practising Aṣṭāṅga vinyasa. There is nothing wrong with this style per se, but I started learning from a video, which meant that I found it difficult to set my own pace. I suffered from extreme heat and insomnia for quite a while before I understood how to adapt the practice. Vāta-pacifying regimens always emphasize proper daily routines. Regularity helps the body and mind overcome the irregular (viṣama) nature of vāta. This intervention is probably the most important change you can make. It could solve your vāta problems completely over time.
- **Constipation:** There are lots of causes of constipation. We are not focusing on dietary causes here. Vāta aggravation can lead to constipation because dryness (Rūkṣa guna) is building up in the seat of vāta, the colon. Stress, pharmaceutical drugs and a low-fibre diet should be cancelled out as causative factors first. It is also unwise to exercise too close to mealtimes.
- **Exhaustion:** If you want to lie down and go to sleep after your yoga practice, you are probably overdoing it. When you start to pacify vāta regularly, your parasympathetic nervous system kicks in and your body takes full advantage by trying to rest whenever it can, even in a yoga class. This kind of tiredness comes because you have worn yourself out. When we are emotionally unwell, we can get into cycles of overdoing, leading to exhaustion, and then doing the whole thing all over again once we have recovered.
- **Mood swings:** If you find yourself swinging between extreme

highs and lows, this is another issue that can point towards vāta aggravation. Yoga can stir things up and uncover emotional issues that may have remained buried for a long time. You need to be ready with more strategies for dealing with the emotional impact of change. Keep a diary.

SIGNS OF SUCCESSFUL PRACTICE

- **Freedom of movement:** Your body feels free to express itself however it wants. There is no stiffness stopping you bending down to pick something up, twisting round to say hello to someone you recognize, looking up at the stars, reaching up to get something off the top shelf, bending back and opening your arms to the wind and so on. There is no reason why you shouldn't be able to regain this ability, even as you age.
- **A steady and stable body:** If you have been suffering from twitches, shakes and unsteadiness, a well-designed vāta practice should help you overcome that. You will need to concentrate on steady holds, steady breathing and mental focus. This should help you build a strong and stable body.
- **Feeling grounded:** As an extension to that, if the light quality of vāta has made you feel very ungrounded, a proper vāta practice will help to root you. That unsettled, flighty quality will begin to subside, and you will build up more steadiness both physically and psychologically.
- **Normal digestion and good sleep:** If you can maintain a harmonious flow in the five vayus, this should help you to rekindle your agni, to rebalance pitta and kapha so your body is able to return to a state of normality.

VĀTA SEQUENCE

In consideration of the above, a Vāta sequence (see Appendix 2) will include:

- A gentle approach that starts dynamically but gradually moves towards greater stillness
- Careful integration of a smooth, deep and even ujjayi breath
- A focus on bring energy and awareness to the 'vāta band', which includes the colon, hips, pelvis, bladder, lower back and kidneys
- Consideration of the organs and tissues that have a resonance with vāta, including the bones, joints, spine, nervous system, mind and senses.

SUBTLE PRACTICES FOR HARMONIZING VĀTA

Vāta is subtle in essence because it is formed with air and space. The essence of vāta is prāṇa, and practices that involve the manipulation of prāṇa need to be approached with care. This is because prāṇa can easily turn into vāta and end up aggravating existing vāta even more.

Here are the subtle techniques that are useful for managing Vāta.

- **Anuloma Viloma:** Loosely translated as 'alternate nostril breathing', this term actually means 'flow and counterflow'. In many traditions, it is also called 'Nādi Śodhana', but in this context the former is more appropriate because we want to use the practice to balance the flow of vāta. The word 'anuloma' means 'right direction' and in Āyurvedic texts, it usually refers to one of the five vayus or five winds of vāta. Anuloma Viloma helps to balance the relationship between the two primary flows of vāta: prāṇa, associated with the inhalation, and apāna, with the exhalation. When we balance the *in* breath and the *out* breath, this can help to balance vāta overall and we begin to feel calm, balanced and centred, our natural state. For general practice, it is best to work with an even ratio of 4:4:4:4, but ratios can be changed for therapeutic purposes (e.g., a longer exhalation will help to bring an aggravated vāta down much faster).
- **Yoga Nidrā:** This is a very powerful technique for balancing Vāta. It is best done during vāta time, between 4pm and 6pm.
- **Mindful breathing:** A very simple practice that is best done after

āsana. It would be very difficult to do it before if you are very vāta aggravated, because it will be impossible to sit still.

- **Walking meditation:** A great way for a vāta-aggravated person to work with the mind is by learning how to coordinate mindful walking with the breath: 3–4 steps on the inhalation and 3–4 on the exhalation. It keeps the mind anchored so there is less opportunity for it to move into negative thinking patterns.

- **Sound:** Vāta resonates with the ears. Music can strongly pacify or aggravate. Gentle words can soothe, and harsh words can disturb. Vāta is sensitive. Sound can be used in different ways.

  - **Meditating on rāga music:** This can have a powerful effect on vāta. Rāga is classical Indian music that is actually improvised around 12 set themes (local regions vary). These themes can be uplifting or calming. Each performance can be completely different from the next, but the themes are identifiable. Rāga music goes deep. It is possible to get completely absorbed in it as an object of meditation.

  - **Mantra:** Focusing on a mantra can be a very useful tool for anchoring the mind. A mantra is a sacred utterance used to achieve higher states of consciousness. It is an integral part of Hinduism and Tantra and is widely used in temples and monastic yoga traditions. (See Chapter 12.)

  - **Mudrā and bandha:** Prāṇa can be manipulated with locks and seals. There are many ways that prāṇa can be directed. The most common practices are the hand and face gestures. Chin mudrā, for example, creates a circuit that redirects prāṇa towards the body and impacts on how we breathe. Bandhas should be approached with caution. There are many physical benefits to developing and using pelvic floor muscles, and short holds during standing poses can be very useful. However, it is important for a serious practitioner to understand the wider implications of practising them.

Pitta doṣa

Yoga can be used to harmonize pitta doṣa through āsana, the breath and meditation.

Pitta controls all digestive and transformative functions in the body. It also controls all the organs and tissues in the mid-region of the torso between the navel and the sternum. Here is a reminder of its key features.

- It is made up of fire and water elements.
- Its primary seat is in the small intestine.
- It controls the hours of 10am–2pm and 10pm–2am.
- When pitta starts to get aggravated, it spills over into the surrounding organs close to its primary seat. These include the liver, spleen, gall bladder, midback, stomach and pancreas. This means that any therapeutic work around pitta doṣa needs to address this zone first.
- Someone who is pitta aggravated is likely to experience tīkṣṇāgni or overactive agni, which can lead to excessive hunger, tiredness and a loose bowel with undigested food passing out.
- The sub-doṣas of pitta doṣa also control the blood (rañjaka pitta), eyes (ālocaka pitta), mind (sādhakapitta) and skin (bhrājakapitta) so these are where we are likely to see results as pitta begins to normalize.

The qualities or gunas of pitta doṣa are:

- Hot
- Sharp
- Light (solar and weight)
- Liquid
- Oily
- Spreading (sara)
- Fleshy smell (visra)
- Sour
- Pungent.

It is useful to know which of the above gunas are out of balance. Take a look at Table 5.1: What is wrong with me? to see what you need to address.

PITTA AND ĀSANA PRACTICE

During āsana practice, you are looking to cultivate:

- A cool, open and receptive approach. Pitta energy is very hard working. It needs to get its sharp teeth into something and will push towards extremes because it feeds on intensity.
- A surrendering mindset to remove heat and emotional tension. Pitta people are very critically minded because the sharp quality of pitta needs to cut through uncertainties and build patterns and models that it can defend with a passion. Pitta people need to believe strongly in something. There is no middle ground.
- A cool, relaxed and diffuse breath.
- A receptive, detached mind with a soft non-judgemental approach.

SIGNS OF IMPROPER PRACTICE

One of the challenges of self-reflection is that your body and mind are sending you mixed messages. On the one hand, you are feeling freer in your body, more energized and uplifted, but then you begin to feel more irritable. The fire you have kindled is also making you angry, but what do you do? Do you stop practising? This happens with the other doṣas too, and my only honest advice to you is to keep trying to find the balance. It is simply a case of trial and error. Here are the common red lights (pun intended) that tell you pitta doṣa is getting out of balance.

- **Tension:** You're finding it hard to relax. You are constantly seeking intensity through your experiences and finding it hard to 'let go'.
- **Anger and irritability:** You get annoyed at the drop of a hat. You find things to be outraged about everywhere you look. You find moral or ethical reasons to justify your perpetual anger.
- **Fever:** You feel hot all the time. You experience burning sensations around your body especially during pitta time between 10am and 2pm.

- **Obsessive/compulsive:** You get attached to an idea or project and can't let go of it until it is complete, even to the detriment of your own health.
- **Gastric problems:** You start to experience stomach acid, especially after eating meat, wheat or dairy-based foods.

SIGNS OF SUCCESSFUL PRACTICE

- You feel energized and motivated but cool, calm and open minded most of the time.
- You are more inspiring to others than intolerant of them.
- Your digestion is good. Your body feels warm and enlivened but not overheated.
- You do not experience inflammation in the tendons.
- You know when to stop and when enough is enough.

PITTA SEQUENCE

A pitta-focused sequence (see Appendix 3):

- Includes themes around surrender, forgiveness and tolerance.
- Starts off quite intensely but develop into a soft, calm and cool practice.
- Includes a lot of twists and rotations to make sure there is no stagnation around the digestive tract or the midback.
- Includes consideration of the organs and tissues associated with pitta, which are the liver, blood, eyes and tendons.

SUBTLE PRACTICES FOR HARMONIZING PITTA

Many of the subtle practices for vāta will also apply to pitta but with variations.

Pitta is made up of fire and water so any subtle practices that raise tejas need to be approached with care. Tejas is the essence of pitta and if it is not well integrated, it can easily turn into pitta and cause more imbalances. Practices that increase tejas bring about greater inner radiance and illumination. You are literally increasing the light from within. Here are some key practices for working with tejas.

- **Mantra:** A regular mantra practice will increase tejas. It is traditionally taught that mantra is a means to purify the mind or the channels of thought. Tejas does this because it acts as the transforming agent. There are mantras for every need. Bīja mantras are single-syllable phrases that can be practised on their own or used to form more complex phrases. The best mantras for pacifying pitta are śrīṃ, which has a feminine lunar nature that promotes health, beauty and prosperity (Lakṣmī) and śam, which is associated with Saturn, so it promotes detachment and containment.[3]
- **Prāṇāyāma:** There are two excellent practices for pacifying pitta doṣa:
  - **Sitāli:** Roll your tongue into a tube (some people are unable to do this for genetic reasons, so they should do Seetkari instead) and then draw in the cooling breath through the tube. Retain the breath briefly at the end of the inhalation and then exhale through the nose. Make the exhalation longer than the inhalation.
  - **Seetkari:** Slowly suck in the air through your teeth. If your teeth are very sensitive, you may find this technique uncomfortable, so you should practise Sitāli instead. Briefly retain the breath at the end of the inhalation and then exhale slowly through the nose. You also have the option of exhaling through the mouth if you feel particularly overheated.

3 Frawley, D. (2000). *Ayurvedic Healing.* (Second edition.) Twin Lakes, WI: Lotus Press.

Kapha doṣa

Yoga can be used to harmonize kapha doṣa through āsana, the breath and meditation. Kapha controls all anabolic and lubricating functions in the body. It forms the building blocks for growth and keeps the body well hydrated and lubricated. Here is a reminder of the key features of kapha doṣa.

- It is made up of earth and water elements.
- Its primary seat is in the stomach.
- It controls the hours of 6am–10am and 6pm–10pm.
- It controls the organs and tissues in the upper torso and the head. These include the lungs, chest, heart, throat and sinuses. This means that any therapeutic work around kapha doṣa needs to address this zone first.
- Someone who is kapha aggravated is likely to experience mandāgni, or slow and sluggish agni, which can lead to lethargy, heaviness and a slow bowel movement that is heavy with mucus.
- The sub-doṣas of kapha doṣa control the lubrication of the joints (śleṣaka kapha), lubrication of the heart and lungs (avalaṃbaka kapha), stomach mucus (kledaka kapha), salivation in the mouth (bodhaka kapha) and cerebrospinal fluid in the brain (tarpaka kapha), so these are where we are likely to see results as kapha begins to normalize.

The qualities or gunas of kapha doṣa are:

- Cold
- Soft
- Heavy
- Slimy
- Oily
- Dense
- Static (stable)
- Cloudy (sticky).

KAPHA AND ĀSANA PRACTICE

Kapha types usually, though not always, experience poor circulation and flexibility. Therefore, the overall strategy is to:

- Start off gently and gradually build momentum towards a strong vigorous practice.
- Warm up both internally and externally, making sure that the room is warm beforehand.
- Concentrate on heating poses that will make the person sweat.
- Practise dynamic sequences that will keep the person moving.
- Include many back bends that will free the spine, stimulate the adrenals and maximize openness in the chest.
- Practise poses that will kindle agni to try and raise the overall metabolism.
- Practise a sequence that will be invigorating and give the person a sense of greater lightness and flow.

A key challenge for kapha types is motivation. It is important for them to keep their eye on the goal so that laziness doesn't kick in, and if it does, there are strategies for overcoming it. A kapha type can give up too quickly and sink into negativity without giving something a chance. However, once they have managed to get an appropriate practice into their routine, they will stick to it, come rain or shine.

If you are overweight, then this is a kapha imbalance. You may not be a kapha type, so you need to be careful about launching into a kapha type of practice, because you run the risk of aggravating other doṣas. Particularly with kapha, yoga has its limitations. You cannot solve a kapha problem with yoga alone. There must be other diet and lifestyle interventions.

SIGNS OF IMPROPER PRACTICE

- **More lethargy after the practice:** A class should not be too relaxing. It should be demanding enough to make you feel you have worked hard and sweated a little.
- **Mental dullness:** You are looking to increase the clarity and sharpness of your thoughts. If you continue to feel mentally dull, it may be that the yoga is not right for you.
- **Congestion in the chest, throat or head:** This may be more related to what you are eating or how much time you left after eating before starting practice. However, if the yoga is doing nothing to address the problem, your overall strategy may not be appropriate.
- **Stiffness and poor mobility:** If your mobility is not improving in any way, it may be that the yoga you are doing is not addressing these problems adequately.
- **Poor circulation:** If you feel cold in your hands and feet, your practice should be adjusted to make it more dynamic.

SIGNS OF SUCCESSFUL PRACTICE

- **Healthy weight:** Yoga practice on its own is rarely enough to normalize body weight. There has to be diet and lifestyle intervention too. However, yoga can help balance samāna vayu, the vāta that circulates in the digestive tract and fans the flames of hunger. Yoga can also help to maintain good emotional health by creating a deeper connectedness from within so there is less of a compulsion to eat.
- **Better breathing:** When the lungs and sinuses are filled with too much mucus, it can cause breathing difficulties. Shortness of breath may become the norm and the body has to adapt to running on low prāṇic fuel. Proper yoga practice with dietary intervention can help to correct these imbalances and support better breathing overall.

- **Less fluid retention:** Yoga āsana can improve circulation, thus reducing the possibility of fluid retention. Fluid retention may be associated with broader hormonal imbalances, but having yoga as part of a treatment plan can make a difference.
- **More vitality and positivity:** Yoga can help to promote the quality of lightness, which is an essential consideration with kapha imbalances. Over time, you will feel more optimistic and less psychologically weighed down. Yoga can create space both physically and mentally.
- **Detachment:** With greater spaciousness comes more detachment. Kapha aggravation can easily lead to a greater attachment to people and things. Yoga can bring more confidence and a sense of completeness, which lessens the psychological dependency on comforting objects and people.

KAPHA SEQUENCE

This āsana sequence with a kapha focus (see Appendix 4) starts off gently and builds towards a strong practice. You can add more standing poses as you get fitter and stronger.

SUBTLE PRACTICES FOR HARMONIZING KAPHA

The main strategy for bringing balance to kapha using subtle practices is to increase heat, kindle agni, galvanize lung/diaphragmatic action and clear sinuses.

PRĀṆĀYĀMA

Kapālabhātī

Traditionally, Kapālabhātī is listed as a kriya or cleansing practice but in many traditions, when it is followed by breath retention, it is taught as a prāṇāyāma. Kapālabhātī means 'shining skull'. This suggests that its design and intention were to clear the head and create more clarity so the lifeforce can shine through. If you want to teach this to your students, make sure you really understand the practice yourself first. You need to be able to anticipate problems and guide students accordingly.

This is how to practise or instruct Kapālabhātī.

1. Find a comfortable seated position that enables you to lift from the base of the spine. This may include sitting on a block or a cushion.
2. Take a few moments to breathe normally.
3. Engage the lower abdominals to force out the exhalation as though you were trying to blow out a candle through your nose. The muscle contraction should be felt in the lower abdominal muscles. Be careful not to create the action in the thoracic region, which makes the shoulders bounce. Kapālabhātī is mainly an abdominal contraction.
4. After 20, 40, 60 or more exhalations, depending on your experience and capacity, retain the breath at the end of the inhalation and apply moola bandha and Jālandhara bandha. This enables the possibility of retaining and using prāṇa at the end of the practice. Three to five rounds make the practice worthwhile, but this will depend on experience.

Bhastrikā (bellows breath)

Bhastrikā (bellows breath) is thus named because the diaphragmatic action resembles that of a bellows used to fan furnaces. Similarly, Bhastrikā can be used to fan the flames of agni through hyperventilation, thus maximizing prāṇic charge and bringing about a sense of lightness and vigour. As with many practices, Bhastrikā can be done in a variety of ways. The best way to start learning the practice is the method below. Once you have gained some mastery of this method, you can experiment with other ways that involve using single nostrils or extremely rapid breaths. Do not try to teach Bhastrikā if you are not competent at doing the practice yourself. Teach what you know.

This is how to practise or instruct Bhastrikā.

1. Find a comfortable seated position that enables you to lift from the base of the spine. This may include sitting on a block or a cushion.
2. Take a few moments to breathe normally.
3. Take a full breath in as quickly as possible, ensuring that you have filled the ribcage as well as the abdomen, and then vigorously exhale the breath.
4. Do it slowly so you are able to control how much breath goes into the lungs.
5. Start with 10, 20, 30 reps, and a maximum of three rounds. At the end of each round, push out the last breath completely and retain the exhalation. This can also be built up from a few seconds to as long as is comfortable.

Sūrya Bheda

Solar breathing is useful for increasing light and warmth, which can dispel some of the negative effects of kapha imbalances. It is quite a simple practice to teach. Once you have found a good, seated position, gently close the left nostril with the fourth finger of your right hand and breathe in and out through your right nostril only. It is also possible to do this lying on your left side and resting your head on your left arm. The idea is to stimulate the flow of piṅgala, the solar breath associated with the piṅgala nādi or channel that spirals down to the base of the spine. Piṅgala carries tejas, the essence of pitta and, as with everything, is moved and managed by vāta.

Working with the elements

We can usefully refer to elemental symbolism as a way of giving students access to the Āyurvedic paradigm through their practice.

It is universally accessible to students, particularly those who are not familiar with the three doṣas of Āyurveda. Beyond Prakṛti and Puruṣa, everything starts with the five elements. By working with the elements, we are also working with everything that arises out of the elements, namely the doṣas and the gunas.

Earth

The sense of being connected to the earth can be a very powerful tool. It represents our connection to nature as a whole and we generally feel better when we feel supported by it. Most of us live in concrete worlds devoid of any contact with mother earth, so even the idea of a connection brings about a sense of calm and stability.

We can help our students connect to the earth by using instructions like the following.

- 'Give yourself to the ground.'
- 'Imagine you are growing roots through the soles of your feet into the ground.'
- 'Imagine you are sinking into the earth.'
- 'With every exhalation, imagine all the tensions melting into the ground.'
- 'Use the ground to reach for the stars.'
- 'What can you give to the ground in this pose? What can you take from the ground?'

Water

Water has always represented life. It is where we originated from and what we are still largely made up of. It can be a very useful symbol for connecting to our softer qualities, both physically and emotionally. We can help our students connect to the water element with the following kinds of instruction.

- 'Imagine your body is a bag of water, yielding to the spaces between you and the ground.'
- 'Your body feels soft and pliable. You are able to mould it into any shape you want.'
- 'Let yourself go with the flow. Where does the practice take you?'

- 'You can hold a great deal within yourself. You are resourceful.'
- 'Experience the coolness of water. Refresh yourself and come back stronger.'

Fire

Fire is what drives every cell of the body. It is the symbolic fire of life that sustains us. Fire drives our passions, desires and urge to survive. It creates the energy we need to live and to forge ahead. It has the power to transform. Our creative power is an expression of our solar nature.

To help your students connect to their inner fire, here are some pointers.

- 'Decide what you want from this very moment and go for it. No excuses, no apologies.'
- 'Feel the heat rising up within you as you hold this pose more powerfully.'
- 'Use the exhalation to fire up the pose.'
- 'Feel the fire in your belly and use it to take the next step forward.'

Air

Air is the energy that moves through the channels of our body. It is alive and enables us to move from within and without. It is light enough to move freely within us. It represents our thoughts and impressions as well as the air we breathe. We use it to communicate, and the more of it we have, the more we need to connect with others. Air cannot be still. Movement is its very nature, lest it stagnate. It drives all circulatory functions and helps remove waste from our bodies. It is like wind. Here are some useful instructions yo help students connect to the air principle.

- 'Imagine you are breathing up and down your legs/arms/spine.'
- 'Imagine you are breathing in and out of your feet/hands.'

- 'Imagine you are breathing in and out of your eyes/ears/eyebrow centre, etc.'
- 'Direct the breath towards your feet/head.'
- 'Use the breath to help you lift and lengthen.'
- 'Where does the air feel trapped in this pose? Any stuck, stiff or painful areas?'

Space

We can use āsana to help us create a sense of spaciousness in the body. We know we have achieved this when we are able to express a fuller range of movement in our joints, especially our spine. If we are inclined to shut down or clam up physically or emotionally, it is important to engage in practices that keep the energy flowing harmoniously so that we maintain its best qualities. Air and space work together. Air cannot move if the space is inadequate. Pain is one sign that there isn't enough space, so this should inform your practice. It is important to pay attention to where pain and stiffness are experienced and work with postures that aim to open up the body appropriately.

Some students have too much 'space', either naturally or through excessive practice. Too much space can create instability, weak joints though loose ligaments and a greater risk of injury. Too much space may initially appear to be a good thing because the body is so flexible and responsive to āsana practice but, in the long term, it can cause a great deal of harm. Here are some useful instructions.

- 'As you breathe into the joints, feel the space you are creating.'
- 'Lengthen the spine. Grow tall. Make the spine spacious and pliable.'
- 'Experience the spaciousness beyond your physical body. Your energy body can expand way beyond your physical. Make the most of it.'

- 'Feel the space opening up as you let go. Let go of the tension, let go of the pain, just let it go.'

Working with the gunas

A natural extension to the elements is to apply the same idea to the gunas. Gunas or qualities are nature's expression of the five elements. They relate to all the senses and find their expression in all aspects of Āyurveda, including the three doṣas.

The experience of qualities or gunas can be very subjective and can only be known in contrast to something else. For example, there is hot and then there is too hot. What is too hot for you may feel normal to me. There is also the spectrum of heavy to light, for example. A kapha person feels normal and well in a relatively heavier state than a vāta person.

We measure normalcy through the experience of wellness and functionality. If I am unable to move easily because I feel heavy all the time, I will gain more weight and eventually get sick. If I experience so much heat that I am sweating all the time and have burning sensations in my micturition, this is a clear clinical sign. You don't need a doctor to tell you that the gunas are out of balance.

CASE STUDY 1: PITTA

I used to have a very regular student who turned up to every class slightly exasperated, and the first thing she would say in a heavy Italian accent was, 'It is sooo hot!' This would happen regardless of the season, even if it was snowing outside. My Āyurvedic hat was telling me this was a menopausal issue, but as a yoga teacher you can only work with what you are presented with because you are not medically trained. Whenever she was in the class, I would make sure that she sat near the back of the studio with the window slightly open and I would make sure the class was peppered with a few pitta-pacifying practices, including twists, forward bends and quiet, still breathing.

CASE STUDY 2: VĀTA

Tracy had lots of aches and pains and couldn't settle her mind easily. I used to put her right in the front so that I could easily give her modifications and appropriate adjustments, as well as engage with her verbally a lot in the first part of the class. This initial attention helped her to settle. She felt cared for and validated enough to be able to learn how to gradually take care of her own needs during the class. Rapport and connection are very important for vāta-aggravated students.

CASE STUDY 3: KAPHA

Tom sat right at the back and always tried to get away with as little as possible. He rarely followed instructions and his posture work always had a slightly sinking, heavy quality. From time to time, I would deliberately move to the back of the room and continue teaching from there so the back became the front and he would be in the front row. He always performed better with a bit of push.

Here are the 20 gunas again.

Dry	Oily
Hot	Cold
Heavy	Light
Clear	Cloudy
Rough	Smooth
Mobile	Stable
Subtle	Gross
Sharp	Dull

Liquid	Solid
Soft	Hard

The gunas refer to the state of the body as a whole and have clinical relevance when considering treatment protocol. They can, however, also be used creatively when instructing āsana and breathing. The gunas are not fixed states. They are on a continuum that is based on relativity, which is why they can only really be meaningfully considered as pairs. The context prompts you to consider where you might be able to apply your instruction.

TABLE 7.1: HOW TO TEACH WITH THE 20 GUNAS

Guna		Nature of continuum	Teaching points
Dry	Oily	Moisture and lubrication	'Feel your body move like a well-oiled machine.' 'Imagine you are lubricating the stiffness with your breath.'
Hot	Cold	Temperature and emotional heat	'Notice the change in the temperature of the breath.' 'Cool yourself down with every exhalation.'
Heavy	Light	Weight of physical body and mental state	'Your body is getting heavier and heavier with every breath.' 'Imagine your body is an empty shell. So light that it is suspended off the floor.'
Clear	Cloudy	Level of clarity	'How clear or cloudy is your mind on a scale of 1–10?'
Rough	Smooth	Level of refinement of moisture	'Make the breath as smooth as you can.' 'Make your transitions into and out of poses as smooth as possible.'
Mobile	Stable	Movement	'Be skilful and mindful in your movement. Know where the effort is needed and where to let go.' 'Be as still as a mountain and observe your body and mind.'
Subtle	Gross	Refinement	'Refine the breath so that it becomes almost imperceptible.' 'Home in on the subtle movements. Bring the mind into the very tissue itself.'

Sharp	Dull	Focus	'Focus on a Dṛṣṭi (gaze point) and keep the mind sharp. Do not waver.'
Liquid	Solid	Lubrication and liquidity	'Imagine your body is made of rock, strong and solid.' 'Imagine your body is like a bag of water, able to give itself completely to the ground.' 'Your body is effortlessly flowing from one āsana to the next, like water changing containers.'
Soft	Hard	Density	'Can you imagine a soft yet strong body? Flexible and responsive to need like a cat? Can you let go enough to free your body?'

Working with the chākras

Chākras (see Appendix 6) play a huge role in tantric yoga practice but a lesser role in Āyurveda. Charaka mentions the chākras but only in passing as they do not feature in any of the key therapeutic interventions. That said, there are some compelling reasons why I have decided to include them in this work.

- Many of the marma points that run along the front of the body correspond with the chākra trigger points (Kṣetra).
- Each of the seven chākras that are commonly taught (there are many systems) correspond to one of the five great elements, one of the five vayus and an astrological planet, so our understanding of these principles could certainly be enriched with some consideration of the chākras.
- Mantra practice is an integral Āyurvedic approach to working with the mind. Bīja mantras that correspond to the chākras can be very accessible to yoga students.
- The chākra system makes references to many other aspects of Sāṃkhya philosophy, including the senses (indriyas) and the motor organs (karmendriyas).

Working with a new class

We all have that butterflies-in-the-stomach feeling when we enter a studio to cover a class for a colleague or are starting a brand-new class. Hopefully, we will have some basic information about the general health of each student, but we won't have information about the prakṛti of each individual. It is always best to play safe with the unknown, and safe means working with vāta. Charaka recommends that we treat vāta like a delicate flower, and this is how we should work with a new mixed-level class. Āsana work should be conservative and accessible to all until you have more experience with the group. Better safe than sorry. The first class is diagnostic, and you can share this intention with the students. They will respect you for it because you are acting with professionalism and integrity. You will observe all sorts of interesting things in the first class that will inform the way you teach them in the future. Pay attention and observe carefully. You will be a much better teacher for it and your students will gain a lot more in the long run.

Chapter 8

MARMA IN YOGA PRACTICE

Marma points or marmani are sensitive areas around the body. They may be viewed as junctions of different types of tissues coming together. Most joints are marma zones or places where clusters of marmani can be found. Many marmas are also located along sutures, which are places where bone plates merge together, such as the skull. From a prāṇic perspective, sutures create human fault lines where prāṇa can be quite volatile. Other common locations are places where tendons attach to bone or where there are clusters of nerves or plexuses, such as the solar plexus.

A common theme for all marmani is that they are sensitive and therefore vulnerable, but they have great therapeutic potential. They were originally taught to Indian martial artists and wrestlers so that they could defeat their opponents more easily. Frawley, Ranade and Lele[1] suggest that the word 'marma' comes from 'varma', which is a bodily site that requires protection and is possibly also where the word 'armour' comes from. It was developed more fully in Siddha Medicine, a branch of Āyurveda in southern India.

From a broader Āyurvedic perspective, marmani are also sites where the three doṣas (vāta, pitta and kapha) and their essences (prāṇa, tejas

1 Frawley, D., Ranade, S. & Lele, A. (2003). *Āyurveda and Marma Therapy*. Twin Lakes, WI: Lotus Press. (p.7)

and ojas) come together. Inevitably, many marma points share the same locations as acupuncture points.

Marmani are measured in Aṅgulīs, an ancient system of measurement used in India. One Aṅgulī is the width of your middle finger, so its size will always be relative and is not standard. The smallest marma point is half an Aṅgulī and the largest is four Aṅgulīs.

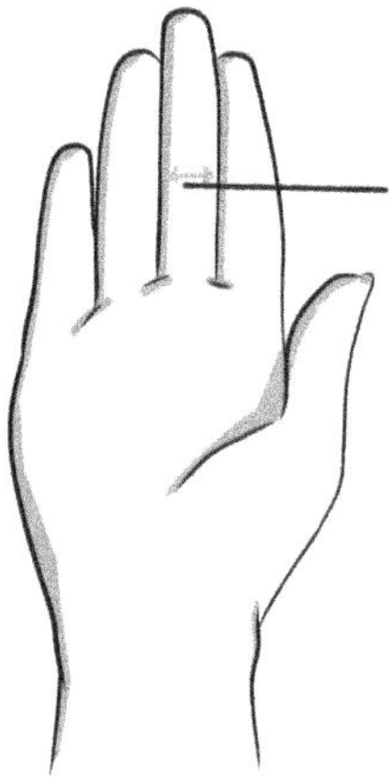

Figure 8.1: An Aṅgulī

Marma therapy is vast and complicated. There are 108 key marmani listed in the *Suśruta Saṃhitā*[2] but Vasant Lad and Anisha Durve[3] list many more.

I do not see any point in replicating the excellent work of my peers as it would not serve anybody. My aim in writing this chapter is to give yoga teachers some practical ways of using marma points in their classes. I have picked out what I consider to be the most powerful points that can be easily located and used in a variety of yoga practices including āsana, mudrā, bandha and breath work.

2 Bhishagratna, K. K. (1996). *Suśruta-saṃhitā*. Varanasi: Chowkhamba Sanskrit Series Office.

3 Lad, V. & Durve, A. (2008). *Marma Points of Āyurveda*. Albuquerque, NM: The Ayurvedic Press.

General benefits of working with marma points

- Working with marma can help to restore balance to the autonomic nervous system, thus striking a balance between engagement and rest.
- The stimulation of marmani can initiate the release of endorphins, serotonin and melatonin, which are all connected to mood, as well as the management of pain.
- Marmani can act like homing stations for information, thus improving communication and coordination between cells.
- Working with marma can expose local doshic imbalances by way of pain, inflammation or swelling.
- Working with marma can help to normalize tissue or organ function by stimulating agni and clearing āma or toxins.
- Working with marma can help to calm the mind and enhance awareness.
- Working with marma can enhance daily oleation routines.

Using marma in yoga practices

There are several ways that marmani can be used in yoga practice.

- **Stretching:** By stretching the connective tissue or fascia where marmani are located, it is possible to release tensions and stiffness, improve circulation and free up any stagnation that may be causing problems.
- **Holding:** During āsana practice we hold various parts of our body to help us create a desired shape. Knowledge of marma points can enhance the quality of contact at the point of purchase.
- **Pressure:** We use the ground, wall and various props to create shapes with our bodies when practising āsana. Direct pressure on

a marma point through the impact of body weight in particular can help to release tensions and stiffness.

- **Meditation:** When working with marma points or zones, visualisation with breath techniques can amplify their effect.

Degree of sensitivity

We have to be gentle with marma points because they are vulnerable and easily injured. Applying too much pressure or stretch or too strong a purchase can end up harming rather than healing.

Local and distal effect

Marmani act on and reflect the health of the tissues they are located in but can also have a therapeutic action on organs, systems or tissues that are located elsewhere. As mentioned, marmani are not only junctions of physical tissues but also a meeting point for the doṣas, especially vāta. The prāṇic body connects the whole body through five directions of movement, which, though seated at various points, create a unifying field of prāṇa that connects the body as a whole.

Another theory on why marmani can impact distal locations is that information runs through fascial lines that connect whole areas of the body. The postural line, for example, connects all tissues that run along the back of the body from the soles of the feet right through to the forehead. Imbalances anywhere along the line would be felt locally as well as distally. A good example is what happens after sitting for a long time. A long period of lumbar flexion often leads to neck ache, tight calves and upper back pain. They are all linked to the same fascial line.

In Chinese medicine, the fingers and toes are the start and end points of the 12 meridians. This is why needling points in the hands and feet helps to relieve imbalances at other points on the meridian that are less easy to access.

Equally, in reflexology, the hands and feet represent a miniature or microcosmic version of the body and a skilled practitioner can often tell you what is wrong just by palpating your feet.

Assessment

Before we start practising with marma points, it is important to locate and assess them so that we can identify any imbalances from the outset. It is unlikely that you will be experiencing all imbalances at once, but you may be able to identify tendencies from the lists below.

Vāta disturbances in marmani

- Pain and sensitivity to touch
- Loss of mobility
- Dryness, peeling or hardening
- Tissue depletion
- Darkening or blackening of tissue, often caused by poor nutrition or inadequate oxygenation.

Pitta disturbances in marmani

- Redness and inflammation
- Hot to touch
- Burning sensation
- Bleeding or easily prone to bleeding.

Kapha disturbances in marmani

- Cold and damp to touch
- Swollen and numb
- Itchy
- Oozing pus or pus filled.

Marmani

The most accessible marmani for use in yoga practice can be located in the hands, feet, head, neck, legs, pelvis and lumbar, so these are the areas I will be focusing on.

I have also trained in Traditional Chinese Medicine and will share any useful information in the 'Applications' sections.

I will limit information about each marma to the following.

- Sanskrit name and meaning
- Size
- Location
- Yoga practices it can be used in
- Applications.

Adhipati

Meaning: Lord, master, ruler.

Size: Half Aṅgulī.

Location: Highest point of the skull on the sagittal suture. The soft spot on a baby's head. This point usually aligns with the tops of your ears.

Yoga practices

- **Śīrṣāsana (Headstand):** A safe and well-supported headstand is the best way to work with Adhipati. Sustained pressure and body reversal have a powerful therapeutic impact on the mind and body.
- **Sasangasana (Rabbit pose):** This is a lovely and safe way of accessing this point without the risks associated with Śīrṣāsana (Headstand). From Balāsana (Child's pose), flex your neck and upper back until the top of your head is resting on the ground. You can maintain this position or, even nicer, roll your head backwards

and forwards along the sagittal midline of the skull so you get to massage all the marma points along it.

- **Visualization**: Imagine a shaft of white light beaming out of the top of your head into space. Feel the connection with the sky and the stars.

Applications

- **Śirovasti:** In Āyurveda, there is a powerful treatment called Śirovasti, where a topless plastic hat is sealed over a patient's head, and oil is poured into it and left there for some time. This has the effect of pacifying vāta very quickly and inducing relaxation.
- **Snehana (oleation):** This point should be included in a daily oleation routine. Rub a little coconut oil into Adhipati every day after bathing and leave it in.

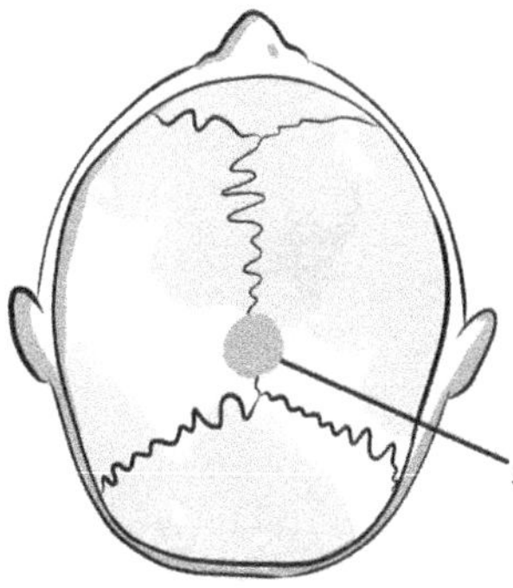

Figure 8.2: Adhipati Marma

Basti

Meaning: Bladder.

Size: Four Aṅgulī.

Location: Lower abdomen. Midpoint between pubic symphysis and umbilicus.

Yoga practices

- Keep lower abdomen drawn in (without gripping) during standing poses.
- Baddhakoṇāsana (Cobbler's pose) can stretch and release tension in the lower abdomen. This is useful for removing stagnation in Basti marma.

Applications

- Focusing on the area around the pubic bone in back bends brings the mind's attention to the Svādishthāna Chākra.
- Use the mantra vaṃ to create a mental resonance with Svādishthāna Chākra when working in poses.
- A warm compress over the lower abdomen will pacify vāta.

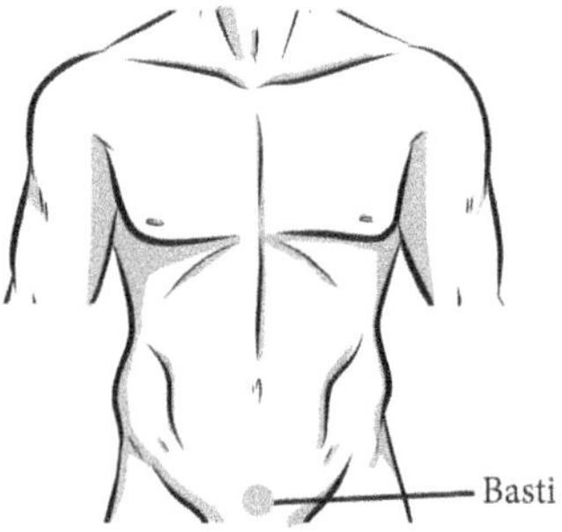

Figure 8.3: Basti Marma

Gulpha

Meaning: Dimple or ditch.

Size: Two Aṅgulī.

Location: Ankle joint.

Yoga practices

- Standing poses will strengthen the ankle joint and improve stability.
- Adho Mukha Svanāsana (Downward Facing Dog pose) will stretch the Achilles tendon and connecting tissues.
- Ankle rotations are good preparatory joint mobility exercises.

Applications

It is useful to include the ankle joints in daily oleation. Circular actions around both the internal and external malleolus will clear any stagnation and improve circulation. There are several useful acupuncture points around the ankle joint that relate to the kidney, bladder and stomach meridians. Massaging the ankles can be surprisingly relaxing and calming, especially when using warm sesame oil and a few drops of lavender or camomile essential oil.

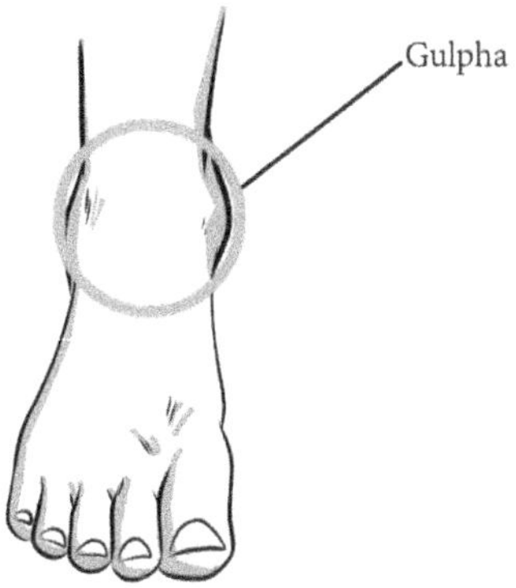

Figure 8.4: Gulpha Marma

Hṛdaya

Meaning: Heart.

Size: Four Aṅgulī.

Location: Centre of the sternum.

Yoga practices

- Meditation on Hṛdaya can help you connect to the emotional body.
- Back bends and Matsyasana (Fish pose) can give a sense of openness and release.
- Quiet forward bends can feel protective.
- Bhastrikā can increase circulation and create a sense of buoyancy.
- Leading with the sternum in back bends prevents neck compression.
- Leading with the sternum in seated forward bends helps maintain length and spaciousness through the front of the body.
- Use the sternum as a gauge for maintaining equal length through the front and back of the body in axial extensions.

Applications

In the context of yoga, the heart marma is the Kṣetra (field of influence) for Anāhata Chākra.

In Āyurveda, there is a wonderful treatment called Hrd Basti, which involves building a ring of dough around the marma and filling it with warm medicated oil. It can be very relaxing and soothing. It is used to ease the heart, lower blood pressure and alleviate angina.

You can also use a warm base oil (sesame or sunflower) and add a few drops of sandalwood (responsibly sourced), lavender, ylang-ylang, rose or jasmine oil to help pacify the heart and the emotional heat it produces.

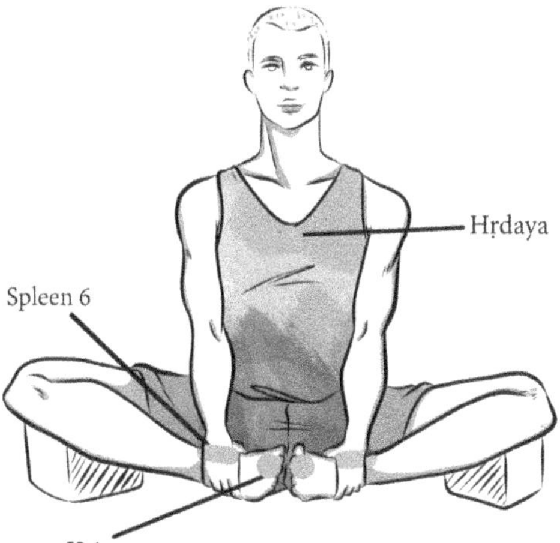

Figure 8.5: Hṛdaya Marma

Indrabasti (arm)

Meaning: Indra's arrow.

Size: Half an Aṅgulī.

Location: The centre of the forearm in the belly of the flexor carpi radialis.

Yoga practices

- **Adho Mukha Svanāsana with elbows bent (Elbow Downward Facing Dog pose):** Press the wrists into the floor and focus the mind on the area of contact.
- **Vrschikasana (Scorpion pose):** Stretches and strengthens the wrist flexors, which become part of the root of the pose.

Applications

Useful for working with carpal tunnel syndrome. Frawley *et al.* use this point to stimulate agni and the digestive system.[4]

4 Frawley, D., Ranade, S. & Lele, A. (2003). *Āyurveda and Marma Therapy*. Twin Lakes, WI: Lotus Press. (pp.106–107)

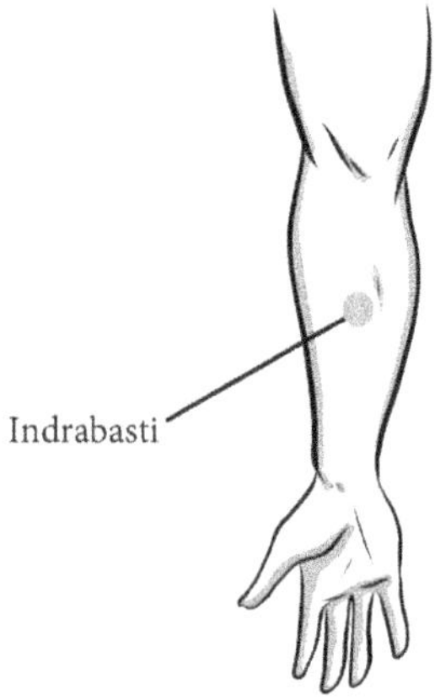

Figure 8.6: Indrabasti Marma on the Arm

Indrabasti (leg)

Meaning: Indra's arrow.

Size: Half Aṅgulī.

Location: Junction that forms a depression between the soleus and two gastrocnemius muscles. Contracting the latter will form the shape of an arrow's head.

Yoga practices

- Standing poses will strengthen the calf muscles and improve circulation.
- Standing balances will improve strength and stability.
- Adho Mukha Svanāsana (Downward Facing Dog pose) will stretch the lower leg tissues.
- Ankle rotations will mobilize the lower leg entirely.
- In standing or seated forward bends, catch the calves and gently press the fingers into the marma point instead of the feet and focus on the point of contact.

Applications

This point corresponds with Bladder 57 in Chinese medicine, which is an important point for treating pain along the postural line, including back pain and cramping. It is also used for treating anal and genital disorders.[5]

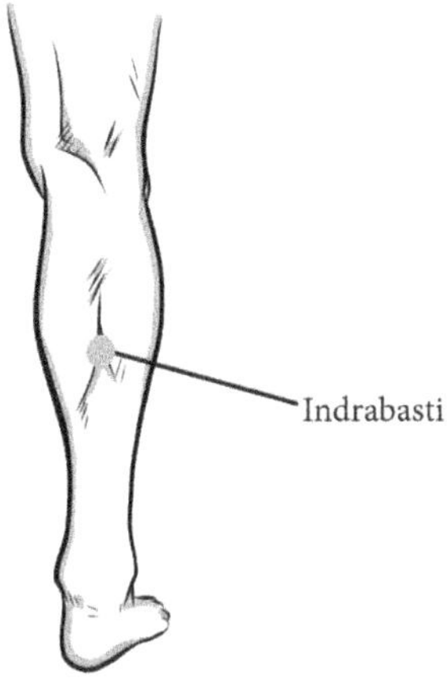

Figure 8.7: Indrabasti Marma on the Leg

Jānu

Meaning: Knee.

Size: Three Aṅgulī.

Location: The whole knee joint should be considered – front, sides and back.

Yoga practices

- Standing poses will strengthen the tissues that support the knee.
- In seated or standing forward bends, wrap the hands around the backs of the knees and focus on these points.

5 Jarmey, C., Bouratinos, I. (2008). *A Practical Guide to Acu-points*. Chichester: Lotus Publishing. (p.191)

- Any pose that involves an external rotation of the leg at the hip joint will stretch the tissues connecting to the inner knee.
- Flexions e.g., squats, Vatayanasana (Horse pose) and Mālāsana (Garland pose), will all improve knee flexion and stretch the surrounding tissues that mobilize the knee.

Applications

There are so many useful and important pressure points around the knee that it would be hard to generalize. If you make sure you spend a good amount of time massaging the knee and surrounding areas well during daily oleation, you will undoubtedly encounter Stomach 36, Gall Bladder 34, Liver 8, Spleen 9 and 10 and many more. The knee is a hotbed of energy that connects to all parts of the body.

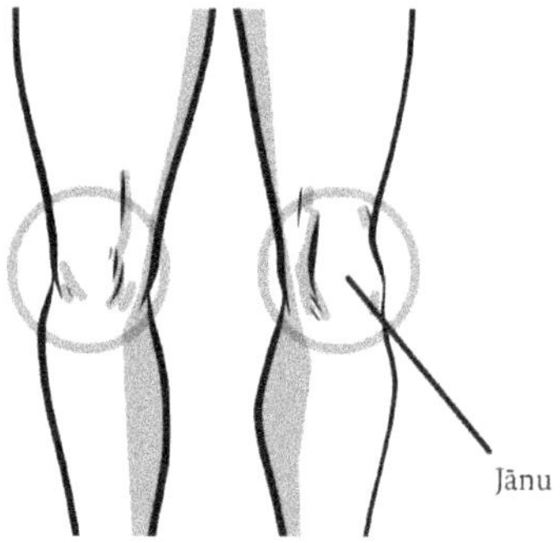

Figure 8.8: Jānu Marma

Kaṭi

Meaning: Hip or waist.

Size: Not stated.

Location: Vasant Lad and Anisha Durve say this is the first posterior sacral foramen,[6] but from my experience it is useful to work with the sacrum as a whole.

6 Lad, V. & Durve, A. (2008). *Marma Points of Āyurveda*. Albuquerque, NM: The Ayurvedic Press. (p.182)

Yoga practices

The sacrum features in all back bends and poses where the spine hyperextends, including standing poses like Vīrabhadrāsana 1 (Warrior 1). It easily compresses with extreme hyperextension and can become very unstable and sensitive as a result. Kaṭi is one of the most vulnerable marma points in yoga practice and must be approached with care.

It falls under the influence of Svādishthāna Chākra, which is controlled by water. From an Āyurvedic perspective, it is mainly under the influence of vāta because it is close to vāta's primary seat, the colon. It is commonly associated with back pain, a classic vāta imbalance.

Applications

- Kaṭi should be included in daily oleation routines as a matter of course because it is most at risk – not only from strong āsana practice, but also from a sedentary lifestyle that includes long periods of sitting. It is one of the key vulnerable areas that āsana practice is adapted for.
- Kaṭi Basti is a wonderful Āyurvedic treatment whereby a ring of dough is built around the sacrum and filled with warm medicated oil.
- In Chinese medicine, the sacral foramen corresponds with Bladder 31–34 and relates to disorders of the sacral, anal and genital area.

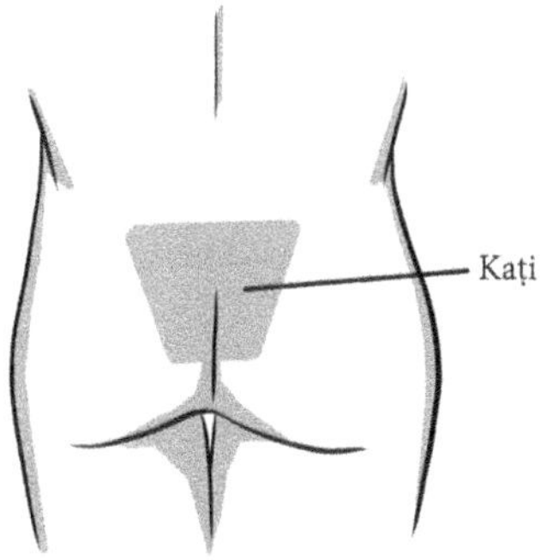

Figure 8.9: Kaṭi Marma

Kṛkāṭikā

Meaning: Joint of the neck.[7]

Size: Half Aṅgulī.

Location: Vasant Lad and Anisha Durve relate this marma to the second cervical vertebra[8] and Frawley *et al.*[9] to the suboccipital grooves on either side of the spine. These are very sensitive points.

Yoga practices

- It is possible to access this point in Savasana (Corpse pose) with a thin rolled-up towel under the neck.
- The same can be done in Sarvāṅgāsana (Shoulder Stand) or Viparīta Karaṇī (Inverted pose) against a wall. Use four foam blocks to practise the pose. Place a thin rolled-up towel behind the blocks so that it is possible to feel a gentle pressure against these points.

Applications

- By gently working with this marma point, it is possible to release a great deal of neck tension, especially if you sit at a desk all day.
- Kṛkāṭikā marma (one on either side of the cervical spine) should be included in daily oleation using a base oil with a few drops of rosemary or eucalyptus to clear congestion.
- This is a very important point in Chinese medicine (Gall Bladder 20). It is used to calm the mind, relax the body and improve vision and hearing (there are fascial connections between Kṛkāṭikā and

---

7 Wisdom Library (n.d.) *Kṛkāṭikāaṭika*. Accessed on 31/3/2020 at www.wisdomlib.org/definition/krikatika.

8 Lad, V. & Durve, A. (2008). *Marma Points of Āyurveda*. Albuquerque, NM: The Ayurvedic Press. (p.131)

9 Frawley, D., Ranade, S. & Lele, A. (2003). *Āyurveda and Marma Therapy*. Twin Lakes, WI: Lotus Press. (p.191)

the eye muscles). It can relieve congestion and stagnation throughout the head.

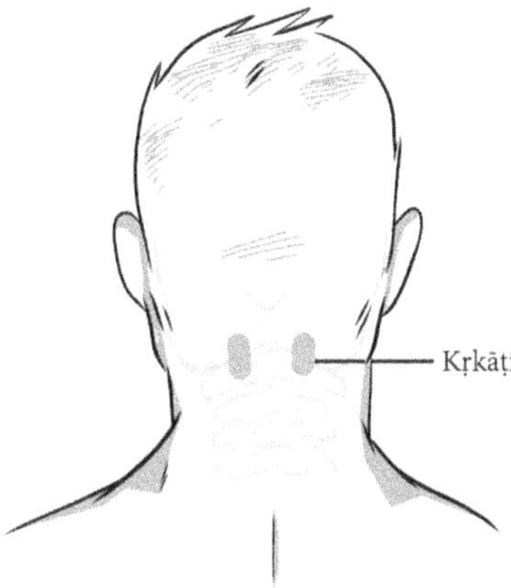

Figure 8.10: Kṛkāṭikā Marma

Kṣipra (hand and foot)

Meaning: Quick acting.

Size: Half an Aṅgulī.

Location: The fleshy ligamentous, weblike structure between the thumb and index finger and between the big toe and second toe.

Yoga practices

Catch the big toe with the index and middle fingers and press against the webbing with your middle fingers. Āsanas could include seated or standing forward bends. Some examples are:

- Trikoṇāsana (Triangle pose)
- Nāvāsana (Boat pose)
- Baddhakoṇāsana (Cobbler's pose)
- Supta Pādāṅguṣṭhāsana (Reclining Hand to Big Toe pose).

Applications

This is a very important point in Chinese medicine (Large Intestine 4). It is used to move chi, which equates to prāṇa, alleviate pain, particularly involving the head, and generally calm the mind.

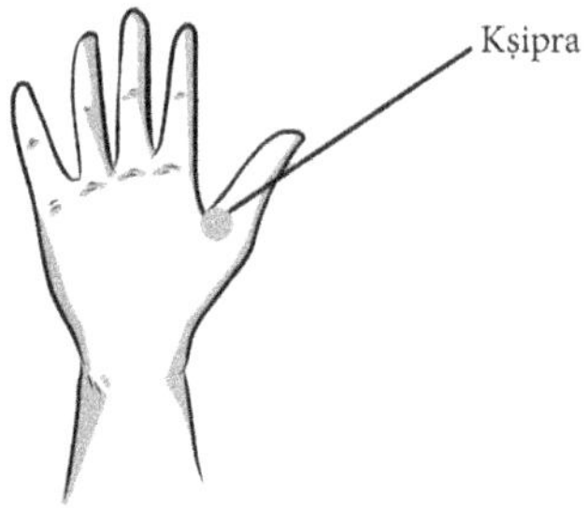

Figure 8.11: Kṣipra Marma on the Hand

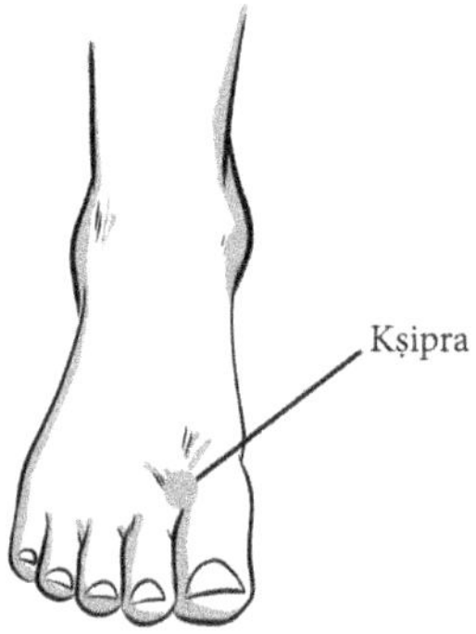

Figure 8.12: Kṣipra Marma on the Foot

Kūrca (foot)

Meaning: Knot.

Size: Four Aṅgulīs.

Location: Mound of the big toe, but its large size suggests that it refers to the mounds of all the toes.

Yoga practices

The mound of the big toe is a very important contact point between the body and the ground when we walk and run. It is designed to take pressure and weight and connects to the entire postural fascial line. All standing poses are useful for strengthening this point and improving posture, gait and balance.

Applications

Good flow of prāṇa and blood will improve the buoyancy, posture and gait for the entire body. Make sure you massage your feet regularly, including between the toes and the mounds of the toes. Include standing posture work in your daily practice.

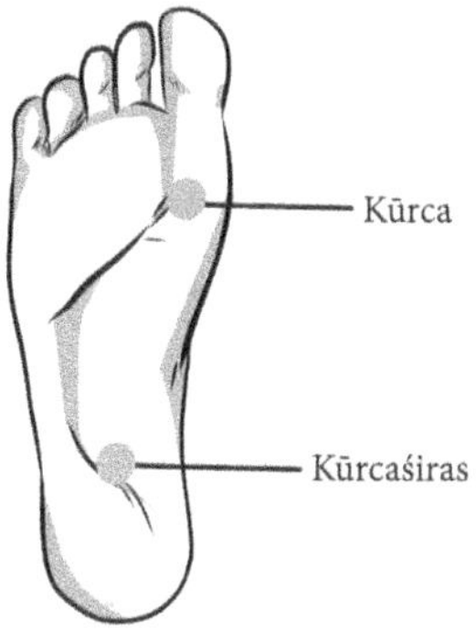

Figure 8.13: Kūrca Marma on the Foot

Kūrcaśiras (hand)

Meaning: Head of the knot.

Size: One Aṅgulī.

Location: The root of the thumb at the centre of the mount of Venus.

Yoga practices

- **Adho Mukha Svanāsana (Downward Facing Dog pose):** Press the hands into the floor and focus the mind on the Venus mount. Use this point to lengthen away from the ground.
- **Anjali mudrā (prayer position):** Focus on the Venus mount in prayer position.

Applications

- This marma enhances the flow of prāṇa and approximates Lung 10 in Chinese medicine, which is used to alleviate coughs and difficulty with breathing. It is also associated with the reproductive organs, which correspond to the astrological Venus.
- Add a couple of drops of eucalyptus essential oil to 5 ml of sesame or sweet almond oil and massage this area to relieve lung congestion.
- To stimulate libido, a couple of drops of ginseng or ylang-ylang essential oil can be used.
- To calm the mind and settle prāṇa, use lavender oil.

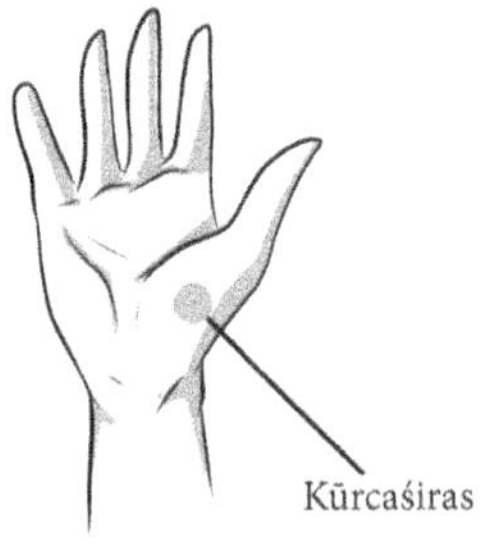

Figure 8.14: Kūrcaśiras Marma on the Hand

Kūrcaśiras (foot)

Meaning: Head of the knot.

Size: One Aṅgulī.

Location: Heel bone. Midpoint of the calcaneum.

Yoga practices

- **Standing poses:** The heel is a very important pivot point when we walk and run. It is designed to take pressure and weight and connects to the entire postural fascial line. As with the mound of the big toe, all standing poses are useful for strengthening this point.
- **Adho Mukha Svanāsana (Downward Facing Dog pose):** There is great value in driving the heel downwards in Adho Mukha Svanāsana because pressure on the heel can impact the entire posture. If it is not possible to make contact between the heel and the floor, it is useful to have a wedge or a block to press the heels against. Caution: The integrity of the spine should not be compromised when attempting this.

Applications

Posture and gait can be improved by working actively with the heel. You can maintain good circulation by massaging your feet as part of your daily routine.

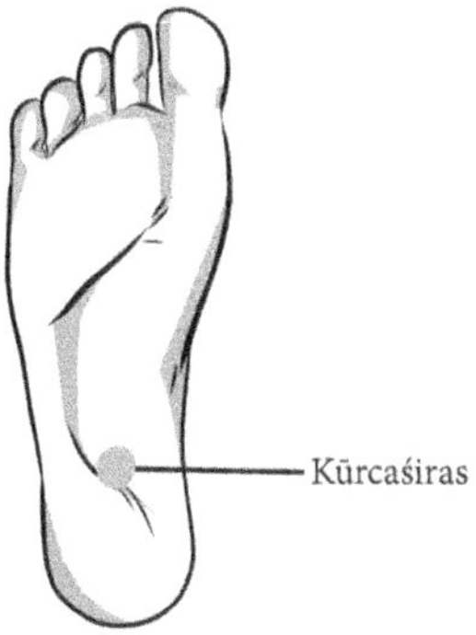

Figure 8.15: Kūrcaśiras Marma on the Foot

Kūrpara

Meaning: Elbow joint.

Size: Three Aṅgulī.

Location: The whole of the elbow joint.

Yoga practices

- Catching elbows in various āsanas, including Parsvottanasana (Intense Side Stretch), Śīrṣāsana (Headstand) and arms above the head.
- Makarasana (Crocodile pose) to strengthen the joint.

Applications

Pressing against the end of the outer crease of the elbow (Large Intestine 11) will release excess heat and cool the body down. It is also used to expel excess wind or vāta and drain damp. It has also been used clinically to relieve abdominal pain and distension and other digestive problems.[10]

It is helpful to massage a few drops of sandalwood essential oil (responsibly sourced) mixed in base oil into the whole elbow joint to help cool the body and calm the mind.

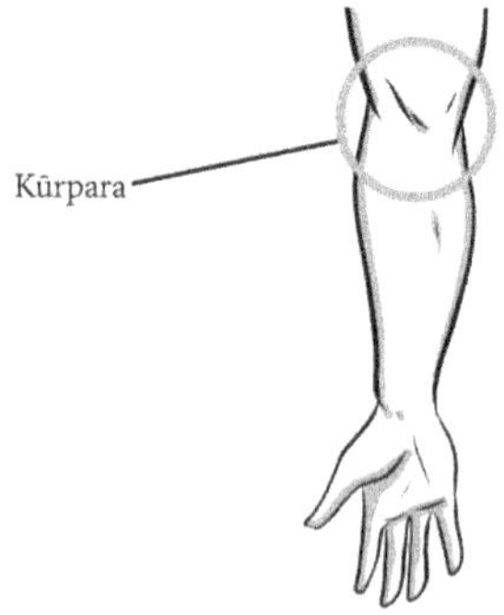

Figure 8.16: Kūrpara Marma

10 Lad, V. & Durve, A. (2008). *Marma Points of Āyurveda*. Albuquerque, NM: The Ayurvedic Press. (p.196)

Lohitākṣa (also known as Kaksha, which means 'armpit')

Meaning: Red-eyed (Vishnu).[11]

Size: Half an Aṅgulī.

Location: Centre of the armpit (axillary artery).

Yoga practices

- **Padahirasana[12] (Bihar School of Yoga practice):** Sit in a kneeling position. Cross the arms in front of the chest and place the hands inside the opposite armpits with the thumbs pointing upwards. Breathe slowly and evenly until the flow of breath becomes equalized in both nostrils. The same pressure can be applied with a T-shaped stick (Danda) until the breath is equalized.
- You can unblock the right nostril by lying on your left side over your left arm and placing your right fist inside your left armpit and vice versa.

Applications

- Lohitākṣa corresponds to Heart 1 in Chinese medicine, which is a very useful and useable point in yoga. There are many lymph nodes in this area, so it promotes drainage. It is normal for this point to be a little tender. Any swelling or inflammation suggests that the immune system has been activated.
- There is a similar point lateral to the pubic bone through which the femoral artery passes. This is also known as Lohitākṣa and is

---

11 Wisdom Library (n.d.) *Vishnu*. Accessed on 31/3/2021 at www.wisdomlib.org/definition/lohitaksha.

12 Satyananda Saraswati, Swami (1997) *Āsana, Prāṇāyāma, Mudrā, Bandha*. Bihar: Bihar School of Yoga. (p.112)

used to balance inguinal glands, but it is not that easy for yoga practitioners to locate.

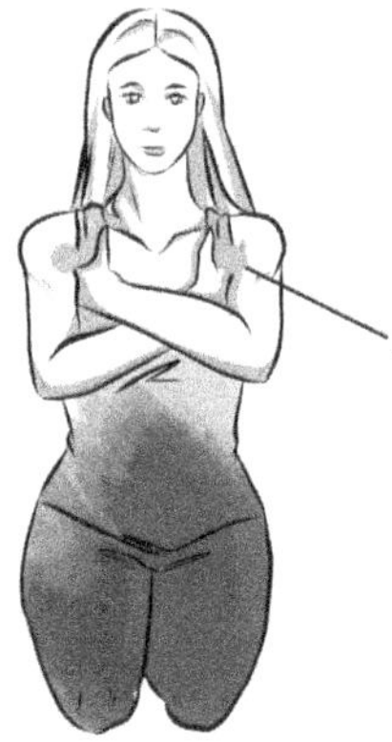

Figure 8.17: Lohitākṣa Marma

Māṇibandha

Meaning: Wrist or fastening of jewels.[13]

Size: Two Aṅgulī.

Location: The centre of the wrist crease, spanning two Aṅgulī.

Yoga practices

- **Adho Mukha Svanāsana (Downward Facing Dog pose):** Press the hands into the floor and focus the mind on the Venus mount. Use this point to lengthen away from the ground.
- **Anjali mudrā (prayer position):** Focus on the Venus mount in prayer position.

13 Wisdom Library (n.d.) *Māṇibandha*. Accessed on 31/3/2021 at www.wisdomlib.org/definition/manibandha.

Applications

There are differing opinions on exactly where this point is, and this could be because there are several acupuncture points along the wrist crease that are connected to different meridians. For our purposes, it is best to consider the whole length of the wrist crease as potentially therapeutic and worthy of attention. The very centre of the crease corresponds to Pericardium 7, which addresses emotional disturbance. Vasant Lad and Anisha Durve use this point to treat haemorrhoids and imbalances in the reproductive system.[14]

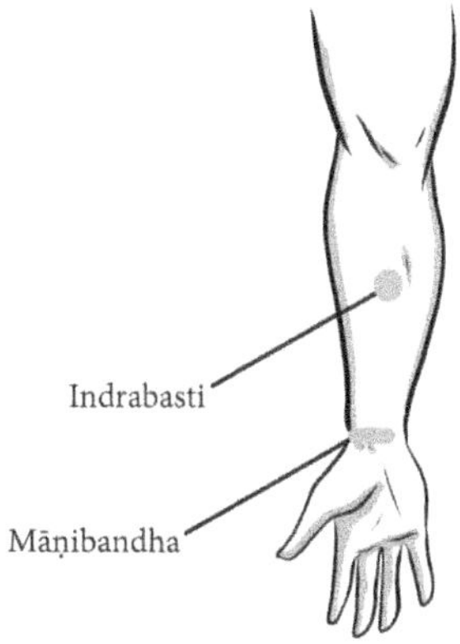

Figure 8.18: Māṇibandha Marma

Nābhi

Meaning: Centre. Focal point. Nave (of a wheel).

Size: Four Aṅgulī.

Location: Umbilicus and surrounding area.

14 Lad, V. & Durve, A. (2008). *Marma Points of Āyurveda.* Albuquerque, NM: The Ayurvedic Press. (p.200)

Yoga practices

- **Agni Sara:** A pumping action that focuses on the Nābhi to stimulate agni.
- **Kapālabhātī:** Repeated forced exhalations done quickly through the nose as a pumping action.
- **Twists, back bends and forward bends:** These will stretch, squeeze, tone and compress the tissues connected to the Nābhi.

Applications

The umbilicus is a very sensitive marma point so should not be prodded and poked too much. It is better to work around the umbilicus when oiling the body rather than work with it directly. Massage in a clockwise direction using a base oil of sesame with a couple of drops of ginger essential oil added. Alternative oils are rosemary and black pepper.

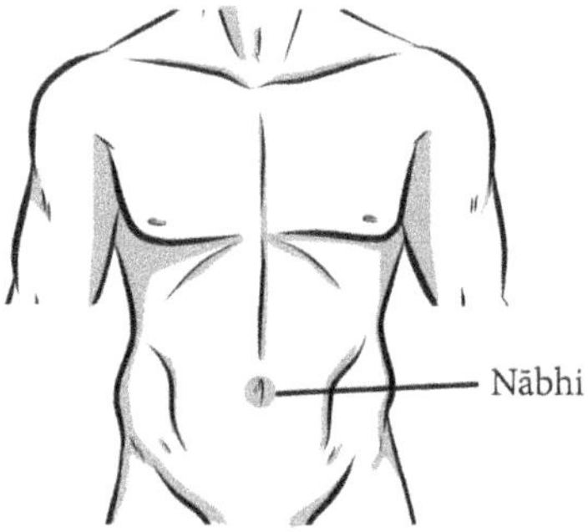

Figure 8.19: Nābhi Marma

Nāsā Agra

Meaning: Nose tip.

Size: Half Aṅgulī.

Location: Tip of nose.

Yoga practices

- **Nāsikāgra mudrā:** Roll your eyes downwards and inwards and focus on the nose tip during an inhaled retention (but not after an exhalation). It connects to and helps awaken Mūlādhāra Chākra. It helps calm the mind and dispel anger.
- **Visualization:** Breathe mindfully using the ujjayi breath whilst focusing the mind on the nose tip. Imagine you are breathing up and down the bridge of the nose between the nose tip and the eyebrow centre.

Applications

- **Oleation:** Rub the nose tip very gently using just one or two drops of essential oil in 5 ml of base oil. The nose tip is very sensitive so don't press too hard. You can use the following oils as suggestions.
  - **Eucalyptus:** To decongest the lungs and sinuses.
  - **Lavender:** To calm the mind.
  - **Clary sage:** To clear the mind and uplift your mood.
  - **Rosemary:** To uplift you and raise your spirits.
  - **Basil:** To help you deal with emotional stress.
  - **Ginger:** To help clear your head.

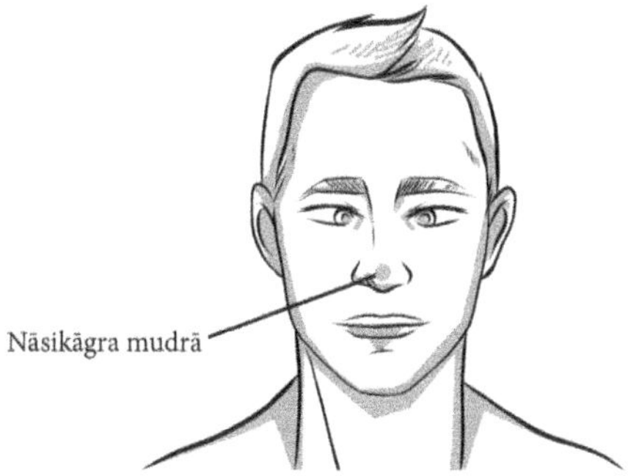

Figure 8.20: Nāsikāgra Mudrā and Nāsā Agra Marma

Śaṅkha

Meaning: Conch.

Size: Half Aṅgulī.

Location: Temples.

Yoga practices

- The best practice for working with Śaṅkha is Savasana (Corpse pose) using an eye bag. Many eye bags will reach as far as the temples, so a very light pressure can be therapeutic. A lavender-scented eye bag would be even better.
- Rub your hands together vigorously and, instead of placing them over your eyes, cup your temples.
- Plug your ears with your thumbs, make a gentle fist with the other fingers and place the fists over your temples. Then, practise Brmhari (humming bee breath) three times, feeling the resonance around your temples.

Applications

Your temples are very sensitive and injury can easily lead to a loss of consciousness, so any therapeutic work needs to be approached with care. I would only use a very gentle oil for the temples, perhaps just one drop of lavender in base oil, otherwise you can easily end up with a headache. Śaṅkha should be included in your daily oleation, but only for a few seconds. In Chinese medicine, this point is used for headaches, eye disorders and pain and swelling in the face.

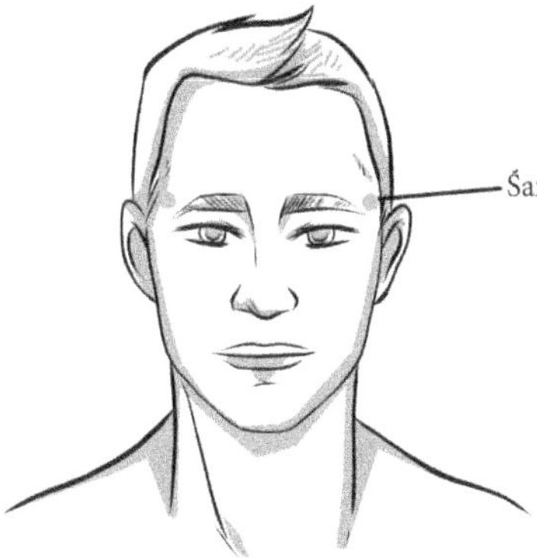

Figure 8.21: Śaṅkha Marma

Śṛṅgāṭaka

Meaning: Place where four roads meet.

Size: Four Aṅgulī.

Location: Meeting point between the channels of the ears (Eustachian tubes), nose and throat. The tear ducts drain into the nose, which also connects to the back of the throat, so it is connected to all the major sense organs in the head. The point itself starts at the soft palate and works its way back towards Vishuddhi Chākra.

Yoga practices

- **Khechari mudrā:** This is the main practice to access Śṛṅgāṭaka. Fold your tongue back until the tip is able to touch the soft palate, and hold it there as you focus the mind and breath on that point. A fuller expression of this mudrā involves cutting the frenulum so that the tongue can be fully immersed in the marma, but this is neither recommended nor desirable.
- **Nada yoga (sound yoga):** Blocking the ears and focusing on inner sounds can also awaken awareness of the energy of this marma.
- **Unmani mudrā (no-mind mudrā):** Tilt your head back about 45 degrees on an inhalation, fixing your gaze on a point in space at

that angle. Then simultaneously close your eyes and straighten your head, feeling the energy descending through Śṛṅgāṭaka Marma on the exhalation. This is part of kriya yoga practice and can be combined with other chākra work or done on its own. It is best to learn it from an experienced teacher.

Applications

When we use herbs, syrups and herb teas to soothe our throat, we are having an impact on this marma and all the organs connected to it. When we practise mouna, or silence, for an extended period of time, this can give time for healing after a period of sensory exhaustion, and the brightness in our eyes soon returns.

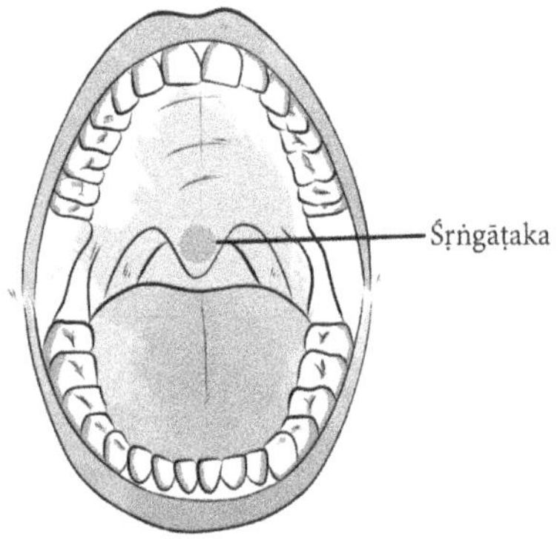

Figure 8.22: Śṛṅgāṭaka Marma

Sthāpanī

Meaning: What gives support.

Size: Half Aṅgulī.

Location: Between the eyebrows (junction of the glabella and two nasal bones).

Yoga practices

- **Meditation:** Sthāpanī is the Kṣetra (field of influence) for Ājñā Chākra, which is located in the pituitary gland, so meditating on Sthāpanī creates a resonance with Ājñā. This point is commonly used to cultivate stable attention during meditation.
- **Moisture:** Beginners can rub a little saliva on Sthāpanī to help sustain focus during practice.
- **Dhāraṇā:** Another way to use this point is to imagine you are breathing in and out of it and use the breath as your focus.
- **Shambhavi mudrā:** Roll your eyes upwards and inwards and focus on the eyebrow centre for the course of an inhalation and then relax the eyes and exhale slowly.
- **Vṛkṣāsana (Tree pose):** Imagine you are gazing through the eyebrow centre as you hold your attention on a single point ahead of you.
- **Savasana (Corpse pose) using eye bags:** Rest the eye bag over your forehead and focus on the eyebrow centre during relaxation.
- **Shanmukhi mudrā (closing the seven gates):** Block your ears (two gates) with your thumbs, and use your fourth fingers to close your nostrils (two gates) and your third fingers to rest over your closed eyelids (two gates). The final gate is your mouth, which is closed. Focus on the eyebrow centre during this practice.

Applications

- **Shirodhara:** In Āyurveda, the practice of Shirodhara is used to calm the mind and pacify vāta. Shirodhara involves the continuous pouring of warm oil over the forehead just above Sthāpanī, which is known as Soma Chākra. It is a powerful practice that is used a lot in clinics to help keep vāta from increasing during panchakarma.

- **Essential oils:** You can add just one or two drops of various essential oils to about 5 ml of a base oil of sesame or sunflower and rub this on Sthāpanī to help cool and calm the mind. Useful oils include:
  - **Lavender:** Particularly useful if you suffer from insomnia.
  - **Clary sage:** To help clear your thinking and lift your mood.
  - **Rose or rosewood:** To calm the mind and lift the spirit.
  - **Lemongrass:** To help lift the mood.

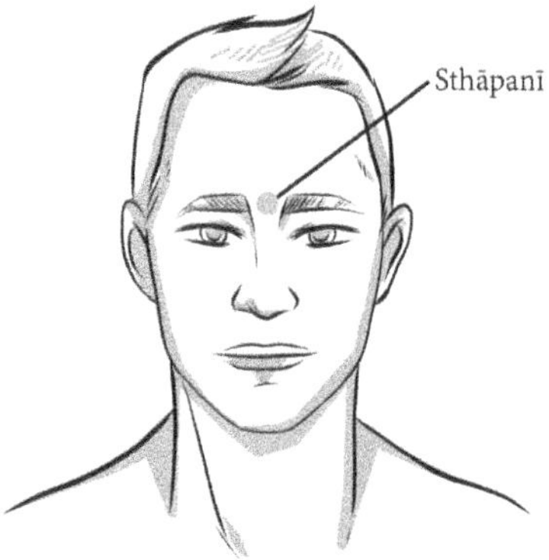

Figure 8.23: Sthāpanī Marma

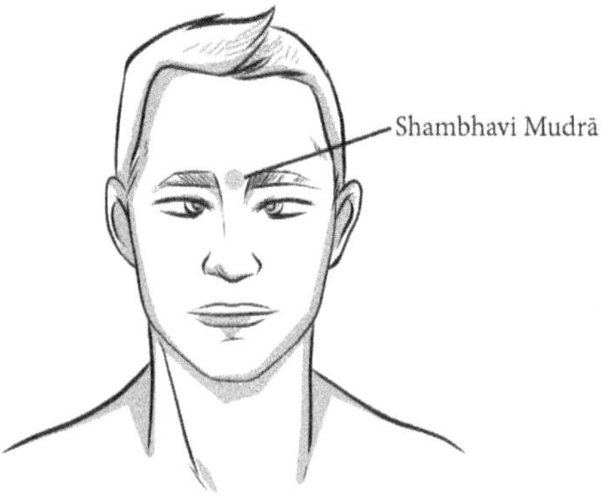

Figure 8.24: Shambhavi Mudrā

Talahṛdaya (hand and foot)

Meaning: Heart of the palm.

Size: Half an Aṅgulī.

Location: A slightly hollow point right in the centre of the palm that aligns with the middle finger.

Yoga practices

- **Adho Mukha Svanāsana (Downward Facing Dog pose):** Press the hands into the floor and focus the mind on the centre of the palm as the hand spreads.
- **Anjali mudrā (prayer position):** Bring the hands together into prayer position and focus on this point as the marmas on each hand make contact with each other.
- Interlock the fingers and rotate the arms inward to stretch the palms.
- Rub the hands together vigorously to create heat and then place them gently over the eyes (one of the seats of pitta doṣa), aligning the centre of the palms with the eyeballs. The same technique can be used to cover the ears to calm vāta doṣas.
- Rub coconut or sesame oil into the palms before bed to pacify the doṣas.
- Use the hands as a source of healing energy on other parts of the body or to help a loved one heal an injury more quickly.

Applications

This can be used as a distal point to calm the heart and cool the blood. A couple of drops of lavender essential oil added to coconut or sesame oil will amplify the effect. A few drops of rosemary essential oil mixed with a base oil can be used instead to boost circulation if necessary.

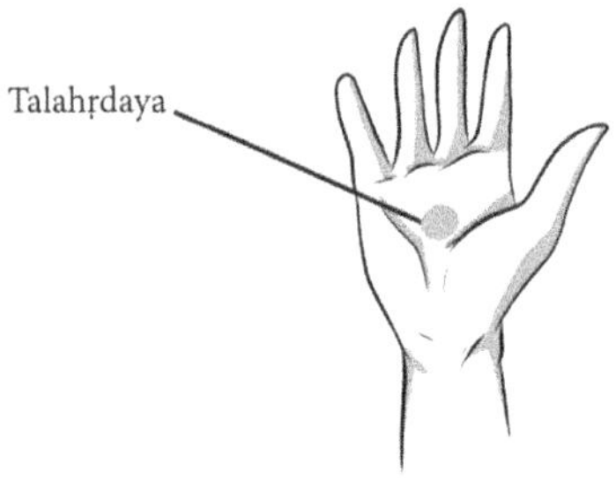

Figure 8.25: Talahṛdaya Marma (Hand)

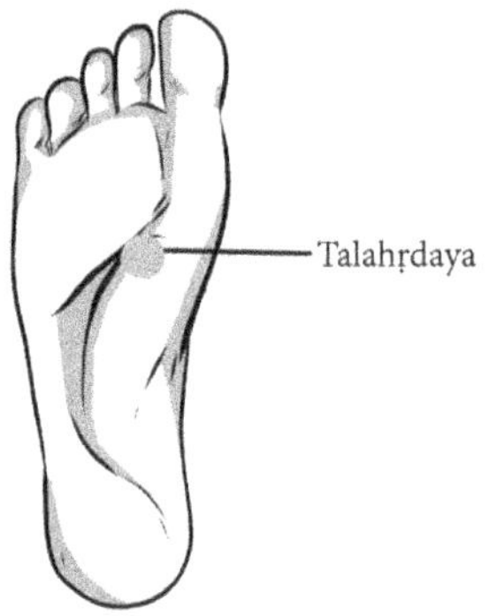

Figure 8.26: Talahṛdaya Marma (Foot)

Vrukka

Meaning: Organ of water filtration ('vru' means 'filter', 'ka' means 'water').

Size: Not applicable.

Location: One Aṅgulī lateral to T12, which is roughly in line with the floating ribs.

Yoga practices

- **Balāsana (Child's pose):** The best way to work with Vrukka (both sides) is to place the palms of the hands over the marmani in Balāsana.
- You can also lie with the legs up the wall and place a soft bolster underneath the lumbar, which will place a gentle pressure on these points.

- An effective Taoist technique is to place your hands over these points in a sitting position, visualize the colour blue and verbally repeat 'chooo' with every exhalation.
- Tone up the area of Vrukka with back bends, particularly Bhujaṅgāsana (Cobra pose) and Dhanurasana (Bow pose).

Applications

It is also effective to include Vrukka in your daily massage routine, especially if you suffer from adrenal fatigue or vāta aggravation. If you have pain in this area, place a flannel soaked in castor oil over the area and keep it in place overnight with cling film and an old T-shirt.

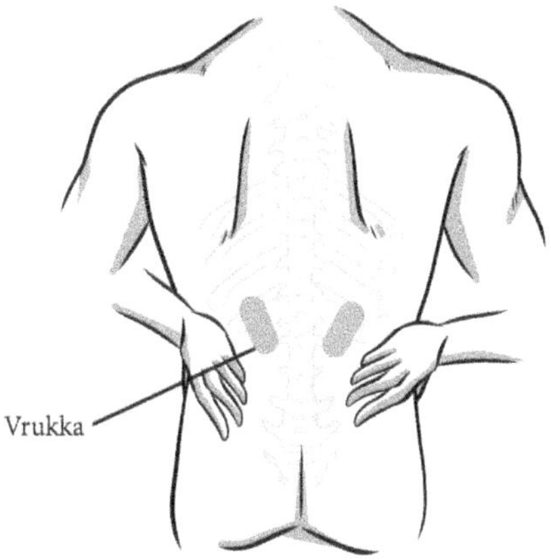

Figure 8.27: Vrukka Marma

How to work with marma points in some key āsanas

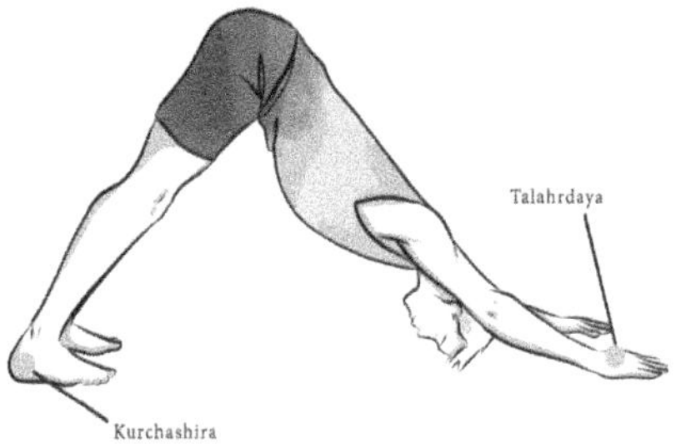

Figure 8.28: Adho Mukha Svanāsana (Downward Facing Dog pose)

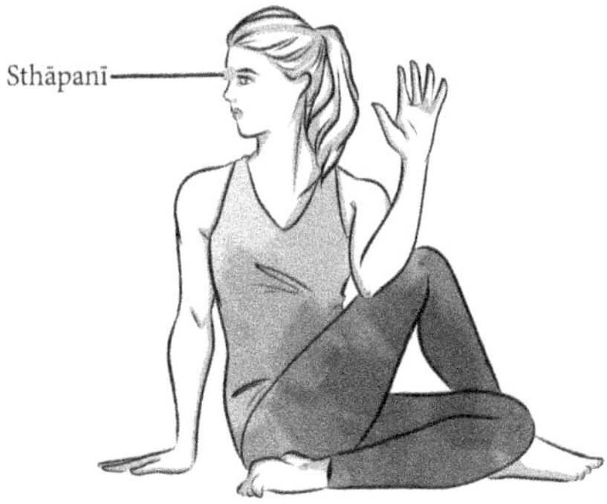

Figure 8.29: Ardhā Matsyendrāsana (Half Spinal Twist)

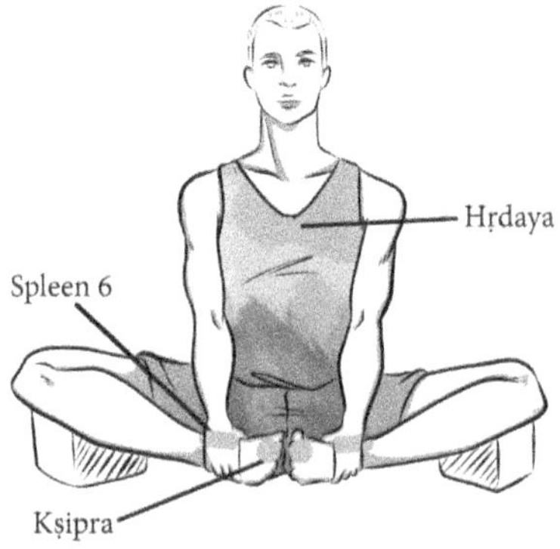

Figure 8.30: Baddhakoṇāsana (Cobbler's pose)

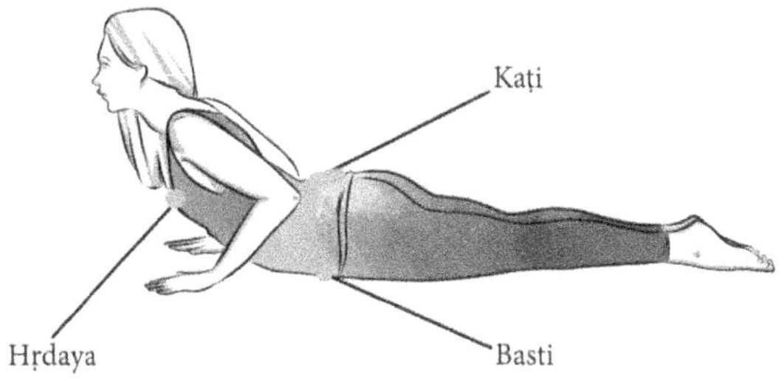

Figure 8.31: Bhujaṅgāsana (Cobra pose)

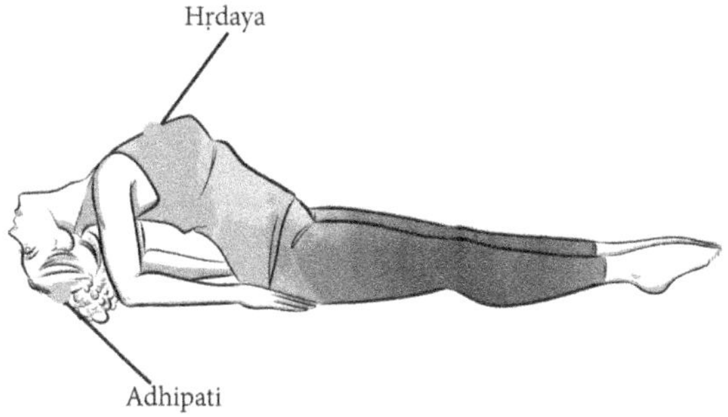

Figure 8.32: Matsyasana (Fish pose)

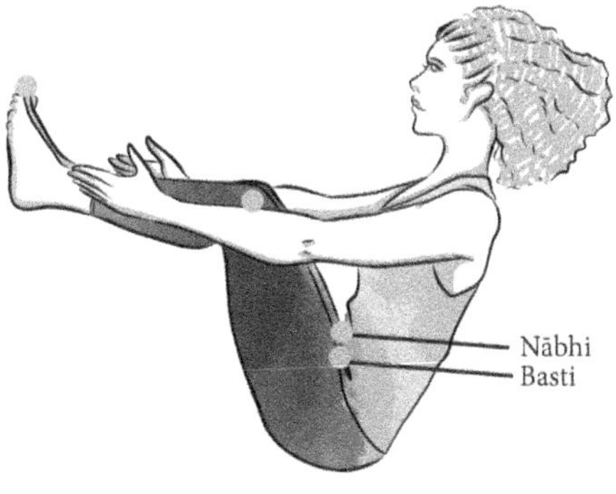

Figure 8.33: Nāvāsana (Boat pose)

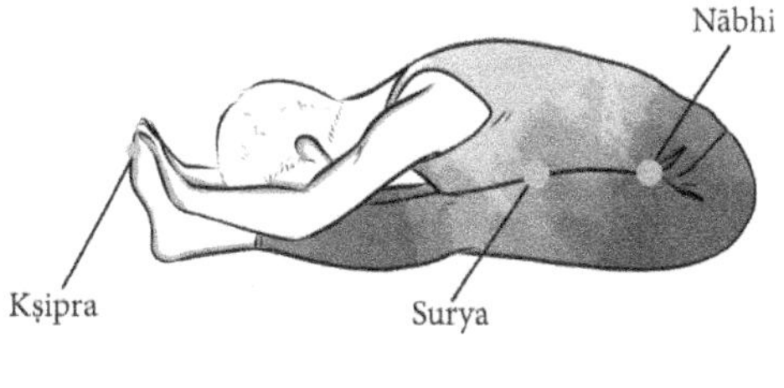

Figure 8.34: Paścimottānāsana (Seated Forward Bend)

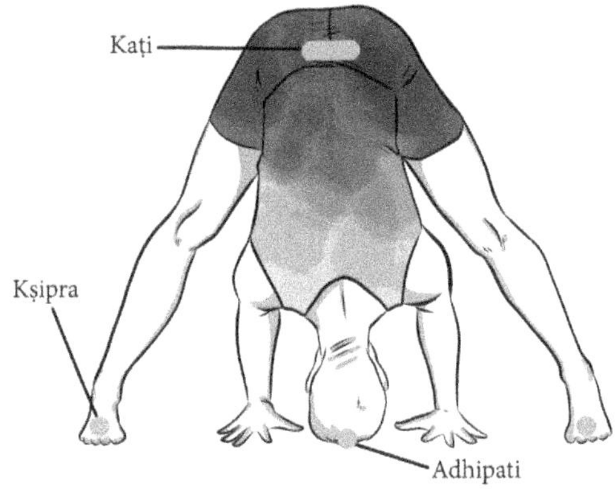

Figure 8.35: Prasārita Pādottānāsana (Wide Legged Forward Bend)

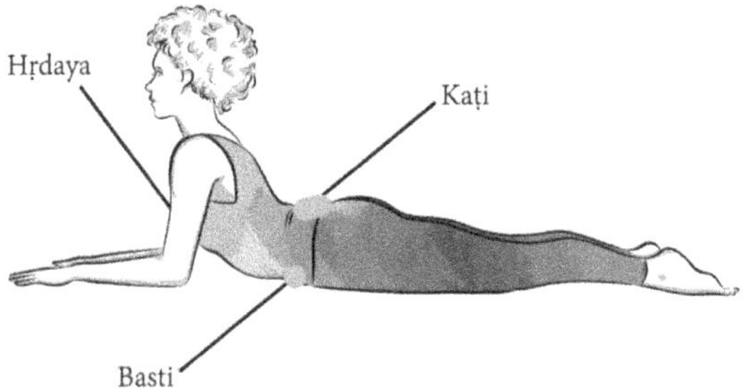

Figure 8.36: Salamba Bhujaṅgāsana (Sphinx pose/Supported Cobra pose)

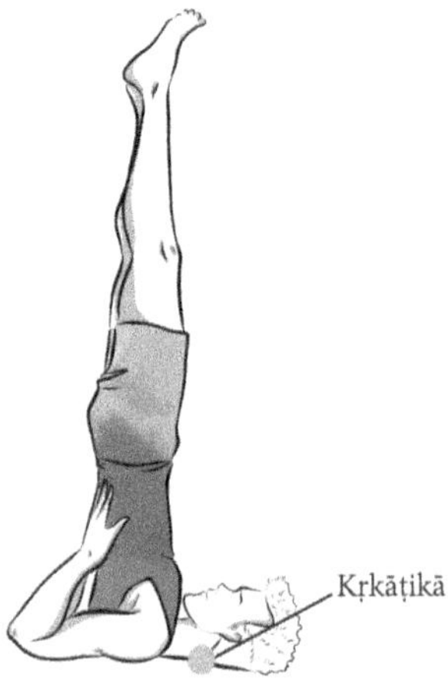

Figure 8.37: Sarvāṅgāsana (Shoulder Stand)

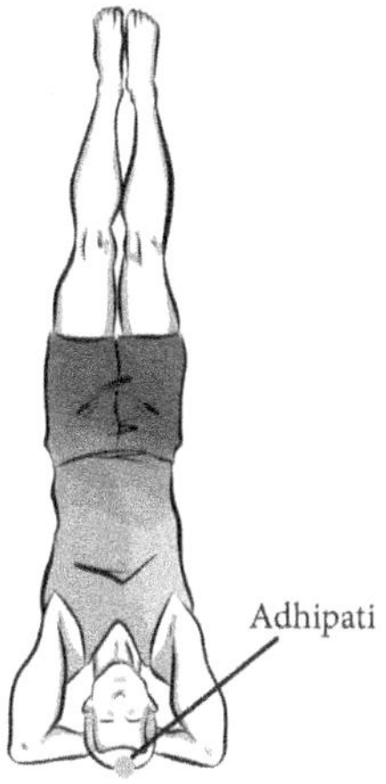

Figure 8.38: Śīrṣāsana (Headstand)

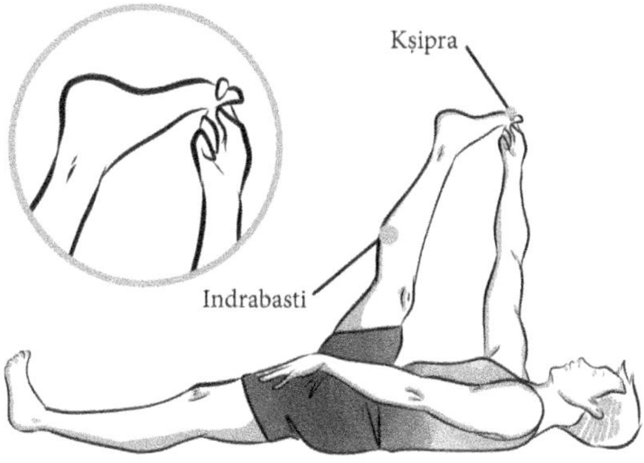

Figure 8.39: Supta Pādāṅguṣṭhāsana (Reclining Hand to Big Toe pose)

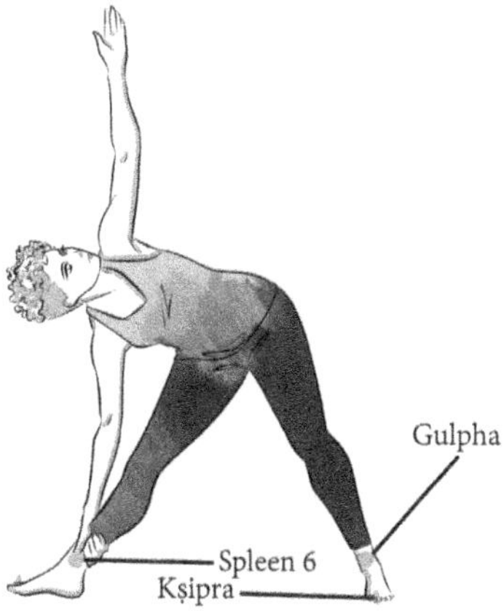

Figure 8.40: Trikoṇāsana (Triangle pose)

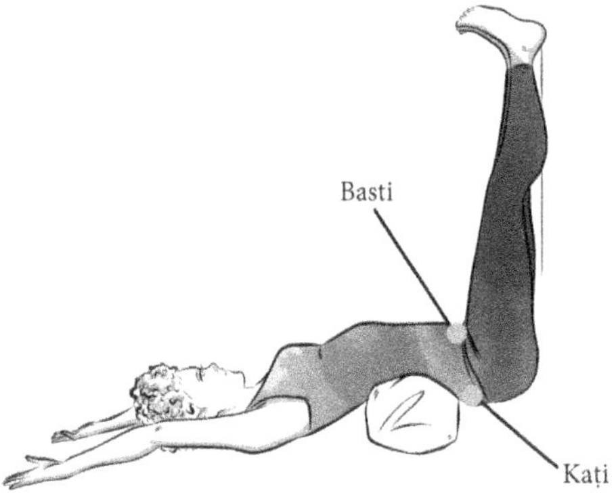

Figure 8.41: Viparīta Karaṇī (Inverted pose)

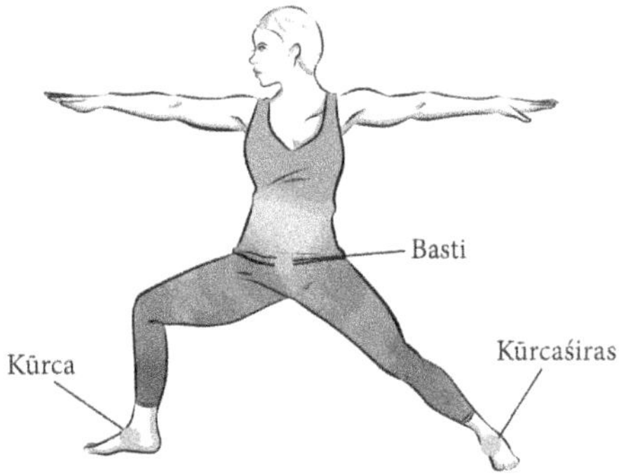

Figure 8.42: Vīrabhadrāsana 2 (Warrior 2)

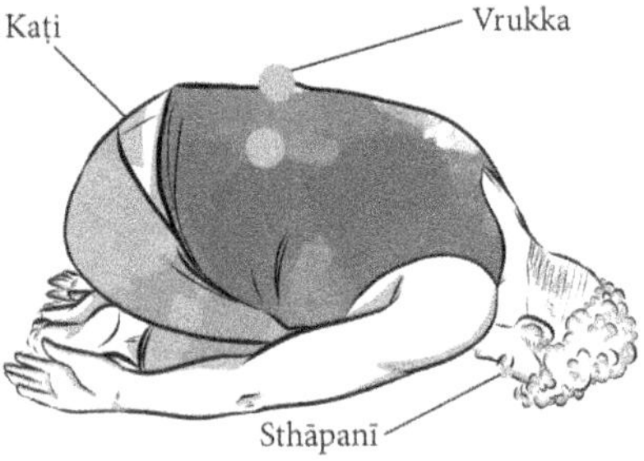

Figure 8.43: Balāsana (Child's pose)

Other ways of working with marma points

Self-oleation

You can use pure sesame oil, any of the oils suggested above or a special formulation known as Mahānārāyaṇa Oil, which is an Āyurvedic classic used for pain and inflammation. You should be able to order it easily online. It is best to give yourself an oil massage either first thing in the morning or last thing at night, followed by a warm bath or shower. Āyurvedic massage tends to work with the grain, so follow the direction of the hair growth (see Figure 8.44).

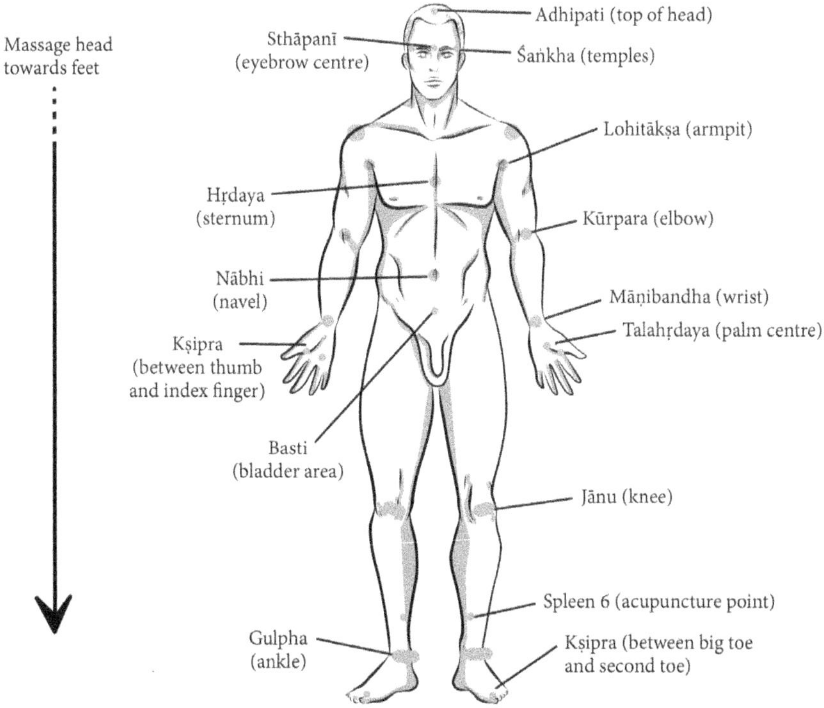

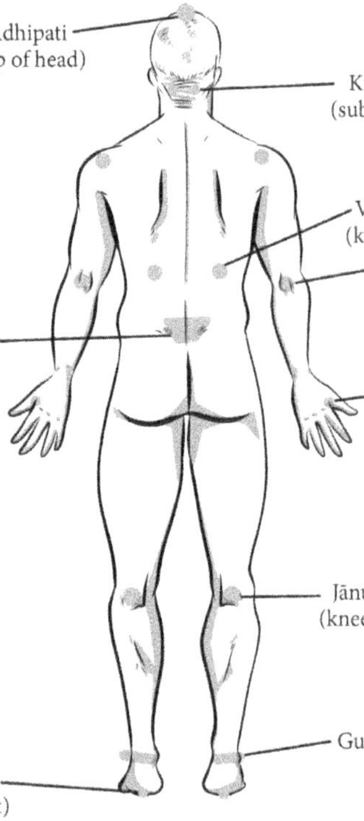

Figures 8.44 and 8.45: Daily Oleation of Marma Points: Anterior and Posterior Views

Hot or cold poultices or hot water bottles

When you have injured a marma point, it is usually very painful and there is persistent throbbing. Putting something hot over it can make you feel worse or better, so you need to test this out. I would prepare a hot water bottle and also get a bag of frozen peas. Place the peas over the injury (indirectly, over a cotton cloth or towel) and see if the pain subsides. It may do for a while and then the treatment stops working, so then you switch to a hot water bottle and see what happens. You can alternate back and forth between the two, and the pain and inflammation should eventually subside.

Loving touch

It seems obvious but rarely gets a mention in Āyurveda books: a loving and healing touch can be the most powerful healer of all. You can do away with your crystals, lotions and potions if you are lucky enough to be receiving loving touch. Healing energy becomes much more effective when it is targeted at marmani. A healer who understands the energy body will know where to work and how. There is a massive difference between receiving healing from someone who knows about energy zones and someone who doesn't. It is actually one reason why I wanted to learn about marma. After getting a massage or healing from a marma specialist, you never look back, because it goes deeper and the transformation is greater.

— Chapter 9 —

ĀYURVEDIC LIFESTYLE AND LONGEVITY

Rasāyana Chikitsā or rejuvenation therapy is one of the eight branches of Āyurveda used to help the body recover from disease and slow down ageing. Ageing is a natural process, but the diseases of ageing are not, and this chapter aims to cover the key Āyurvedic diet and lifestyle recommendations for a long and healthy life.

As yoga teachers, we sometimes make promises, albeit a little tongue in cheek, that are based on scripture. Indeed, we may even have been attracted to yoga by all the magical and mystical claims made by well-known teachers like Patanjali. I certainly was. Once we become teachers ourselves, however, we are responsible for making sure students are able to differentiate between what was traditionally believed, or at least taught, and what has been verified as true either by science or by our own empirical experience.

Health and longevity go to the very heart of what both yoga and Āyurveda are about. The main goal of Āyurveda is to create a strong and robust body and a clear and present mind as a foundation for rising above our sense of separateness and experiencing the union of our individual consciousness with cosmic consciousness.

There are many outlandish claims made in Swatmarama's *HYP* about yoga's power to extend life and overcome disease. For example, he claims that Siddhasana (Adept's pose) can destroy all diseases and Matsyendrāsana (Seated Spinal Twist) can bring about a kundalini awakening. Such claims are echoed all over the corpus of yogic literature and seep into

Āyurvedic literature too. The *Caraka Saṃhitā* extols the virtues of many herbal preparations and treatment protocols that claim to prolong life and regenerate the body and mind.

The Rasāyana promise

Charaka's Rasāyana Chikitsā (rejuvenation therapy) promises the following.

- Longevity and happiness
- Excellent memory and sharp perception
- Robust health
- Beautiful skin, a melodious voice, kindness and generosity
- A strong body and sharp senses
- The ability to influence others
- Integrity and the courage to hold true to one's word
- A beautiful, smart and youthful appearance.

Fundamentals of Rasāyana

The word for body in Sanskrit is 'sharira', which literally means 'continuously degenerating'. It refers to both the physical body and mental faculties. The process of life can be viewed in terms of losses and gains. During childhood, and up to the age of 30, the gains outweigh the losses because the anabolic process is very active. In full adulthood, the losses and gains are equal (we call this 'homeostasis'), and as we move into old age, or jara, the losses outweigh the gains because the catabolic processes are more dominant.

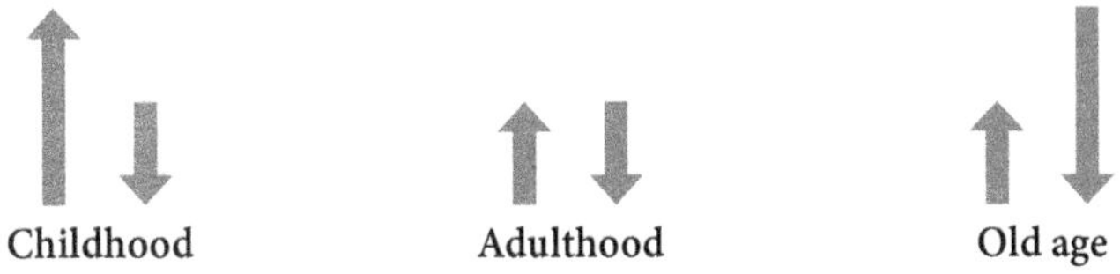

Figure 9.1: Rasāyana and Ageing

Signs of ageing

There are three broad functions that are relevant to ageing from an Āyurvedic perspective. These are:

- How efficiently the senses and sense organs are working
- How well the cognitive faculties like memory and intellect are functioning
- The quality and functioning of bodily tissues.

The diseases of old age are characterized by the qualities of vāta doṣa.

- The skin starts to dry and wrinkle.
- The muscles start to atrophy (light and subtle).
- The bones become porous and weak (light and dry).
- The body becomes lighter and less stable (movement).
- The person is less able to sleep for long hours (light).
- There is forgetfulness and incoherence (unstable).

The two critical factors that need to be managed as we age are a *reduction in ojas* and an *increase in vāta doṣa.*

The negative effects of these factors can be powerfully mitigated if we follow Āyurvedic daily and seasonal regimens. Āyurveda does not separate the way we live from how well we feel. Most diseases do not happen by accident but are usually the culmination of many years of unwholesome living.

We take that to mean that we are to blame when things go wrong, but this is only partly true. Unwholesome living is complex and multifaceted. It is related to our environment, our culture, our economic circumstances and our personal responses to them. We do not exist in isolation. Our world is a place we share, co-habit and co-create. As co-creators we must shoulder some but not all of the blame for the ills of our society. This chapter aims to analyse the various facets related to lifestyle and health, so we can see how we need to act to improve our experience and help to bring greater clarity to our students.

It is worth bearing in mind that you may be your students' only source of knowledge on these matters, so even taking five minutes to sift through the complexities of lifestyle choices could make all the difference to them.

When you ask students about how much agency they think they have when making lifestyle choices, they will almost always say that they are in control of their lives, but this is simply not true. Our subconscious mind is heavily influenced by subliminal messages all around us and only about 5 per cent of it actually seeps into our conscious mind.[1]

What is lifestyle?

Lifestyle is a huge area that goes way beyond the rudiments of what we eat and how we entertain ourselves. It touches on the very heart of our cultural and socio-political values and what roles we play in them. Whether we are conscious of it or not, we are products of the society we were raised in. Our world view is so embedded in the way we've been brought up that we would struggle to remain objective about our so-called choices.

The traditional approach

Providing our students with a simple list of beneficial or detrimental activities taken from the Āyurvedic texts may have some impact, but it may not be lasting or meaningful because the *Caraka Saṃhitā* is no longer culturally relevant in terms of when and for whom it was written.

There is an argument in favour of culturally appropriating traditional teachings while honouring their original roots and without losing their essence. There is no point in retaining the original teachings if they are not able to serve us in the west. Appropriation can be done skilfully and respectfully so the origins are retained but the universality of the principles is applied.

We need to be critical of what we do and how we do it on a daily basis. Without discrimination, we are in danger of following rules to the letter and getting into deep water when things start to go wrong with

1 Lipton, B. (2015). *Is there a way to change subconscious patterns?* Accessed on 31/3/2021 at www.brucelipton.com/there-way-change-subconscious-patterns.

our health. It is important to be able to rationalize why we do things and the impact of those activities on all facets of our being. There are many cultural norms that do not serve us and we need to be mindful of what they are.

Āyurveda recommends certain daily routines that are bizarre to westerners. We tend to value activities that are scientifically endorsed and don't offend our cultural sensibilities. However, it is important to acknowledge that many traditional practices are yet to be understood by science. More and more research is being carried out on traditional methods and a greater understanding is coming to light; but in the meantime, let us trust the wisdom of Āyurvedic elders who carry the testimony of generations of experience in the value and efficacy of traditional teachings.

Impact of Prakṛti on lifestyle choices

Prakṛti is who we are at our best. We have certain tendencies that arise from the alchemy of our individuality and the world we were brought up in. We are created not only by our parents but also, equally, by our society, our astrological blueprint and the environment we were brought up in. We need to consider our innate drives and how well they will match with Āyurvedic lifestyle recommendations. Lifestyle guidebooks are always written from the point of view of the writer, who is influenced by the prejudices of their own prakṛti.

This is important because a wise teacher will empower students to find out why a recommended technique is not working for them. I was once told by an extremely flexible teacher that my inability to do a pose was entirely in my head. I found this incredibly unhelpful because it was clumsy. Years later, I understand that I was trying to mould myself into a version of me that did not honour my prakṛti at all. It was a version that pleased my teachers but didn't bring out the best in me. When you read the *Caraka Saṃhitā*, you sometimes get the impression that Charaka favoured kapha types. His world view was based on the idea that abundance and longevity can only come naturally to a kapha prakṛti. Experience has taught me that this is simply not true. Many vāta types live to a ripe old age and some kapha types die young.

Every one of your students carries a history that must be honoured. They are standing before you because they have survived everything that has happened to them thus far, and their story should be celebrated. Do not use the multitudinous rules laid out in Āyurveda to cast judgement on others. You do not know where they came from or where they are going. Don't be hasty to judge, however much your students want you to.

It takes many years to become a good practitioner; not only is there a lot to learn, but also it takes years to understand how to apply it usefully. The books are the map, but your students are the territory.

> Observe, listen, learn. The books are the map, but your students are the territory.

The scales of life can easily go off balance and identifying the cause is a most difficult art. Create an unconditionally supportive space for your students so that the causes of suffering are revealed all on their own. Your students will experience lightbulb moments and know what changes they need to make. Empower them with the tools from this book so they can investigate their own difficulties. When the fruit is ripe, it will drop off the tree all on its own.

Classroom culture

If you get to know your students, observe them properly and interact with them, you will soon get to know their strengths and weaknesses. You will get to know:

- Their postural imbalances and how they compensate for them
- The poses they like and dislike
- Their general classroom behaviour and the way they relate to the other students
- Their emotional needs and what they are looking to get from your classes.

As you are the creator of your classroom culture, you get to establish boundaries around what is permissible and what is not. It is also your responsibility to feed back to students in a way that is helpful but unconditionally accepting. Students come with baggage and your class is usually an attempt to lighten their load in some way. Yoga is not just about the pleasure of practising; it is a way of balancing the book too.

We often encounter people who are utterly embroiled in difficulty and are completely incapable of solving their problems. However, we often fail to see that those very same people have strengths that we don't see in our classes. They may have a special talent or a quality that lights up a room. If we are strict about maintaining an unconditionally accepting space, our students will eventually show their light. I have regularly been surprised at what my students get up to outside the class. We often forget that even though someone is struggling to do Trikoṇāsana (Triangle pose), they could be flying high in other areas of life.

Vikṛti and lifestyle

Āyurveda describes three different types of imbalance:

- Physical
- Mental
- Spiritual.

All three are interrelated and are impacted by the way we live our lives.

We may be physically sick because we don't eat well or exercise enough. We don't eat well or exercise because we are surrounded by takeaway food shops and we work ten hours a day, so we end up too exhausted to make any changes. We may find pleasure and relief from tasty food and TV shows because we are not motivated by our wider community to act or do any differently.

Daily routines

Morning

1. WAKE UP EARLY

Why does Āyurveda recommend this? There are two types of people in the world: owls and larks. Owls have a lot more energy in the evenings and larks have a lot in the mornings. Owls and larks living in the same household can easily fall out if they don't respect these differences.

That aside, Āyurveda generally favours the larks over the owls because it is looking at the bigger picture. Yoga recommends we wake up during Brāhmamuhūrta, which is a period of two muhurtas before dawn. One muhurta is about 48 minutes, so two muhurtas is 1 hour and 36 minutes before dawn. Vāta doṣa is dominant during this period, so if you can manage to get up before dawn or even at dawn, which vāta also controls (vāta controls the junctions of the day), then you will feel lighter and have more energy. If you wait until after dawn, kapha will have moved into dominance so you will feel heavier and it will be harder to get up. These are the principles, but in reality we are all different. Don't torture yourself if you cannot get used to getting up before dawn. Getting enough sleep is much more important.

2. MEDITATION AND MANTRA (20 MINUTES)

When we first wake up, our minds are still in an alpha state, so it is a great time to meditate. You will get into the zone much more quickly. If you start to engage with people, check your mobile phone, switch on the radio, etc., the mind will switch into a beta state and it will be harder to slow it down again for meditation.

3. EMPTY YOUR BOWELS AND BLADDER

Yoga and Āyurveda recommend that you empty your bladder and bowels first thing. This will obviously depend on the nature of your jaṭhara agni, or digestive fire (see Chapter 6 for more detailed information).

BOWEL DISEASES

Egyptian court physicians used to be called 'guardians of the anus'[2] because, like Āyurveda, ancient Egyptian medicine recognized the importance of maintaining a healthy bowel movement. We need around 100–150 g of fibre a day to initiate the defecation reflex, which is why diet plays such an important part in the health of our digestive system overall.

Constipation or hard stool leads to constant bowel strain, which in turn can lead to pressure diseases.

Take your bowel movement seriously!

4. EXTERNAL OLEATION (OIL MASSAGE)

Āyurveda recommends a short oil massage as part of your bathroom routine.

This is a bit of a sticking point for people (pun intended). Āyurveda is very keen on using oil as a means of controlling vāta because it is the best substance for mitigating the effects of dryness. Oil massaging is less important when we are young and show few signs of vāta aggravation; but the older we get, the more important it becomes. It can be time consuming and the oil is hard to remove once it has been applied. The best way to incorporate oil massage into your dinacaryā (daily regimen) is to keep it simple.

Target the key joints like the knees, elbows, sacrum, lumbar and ankles. These areas have a high concentration of marma points, so they are sensitive. Regularly massaging the joints will help to harmonize the flow of vāta throughout the body. Before you dress, you can reapply a little coconut oil to the scalp, gently rubbing it in. A thin film of oil is enough, and it won't make your hair look greasy. You can also reapply a little to the soles of your feet before putting on your tights or socks. The older you get, the more help you will need, so it is well worth investing in a regular oil massage by a professional.

In India, Āyurvedic oil massages tend to be carried out by two

---

2 Gregor, M. (2020). *Flashback Friday: How Many Bowel Movements Should You Have & Should You Sit, Lean, or Squat?* Accessed on 24/2/2021 at https://nutritionfacts.org/video/flashback-friday-how-many-bowel-movements-should-you-have-should-you-sit-lean-or-squat.

therapists at the same time. Therapists use broad sweeps that connect whole sides of the body rather than localized massage popularized by the 'Swedish massage' approach used in the west. Four-hand massage may not be cost effective when you book an Āyurvedic massage in the UK, but some clinics do still offer it. From an Āyurvedic perspective, it is important to massage with the grain because the direction of hair growth tells you which way vāta is flowing. It is also important to start from the head and work your way down to your feet (see Figure 9.2).

OILS

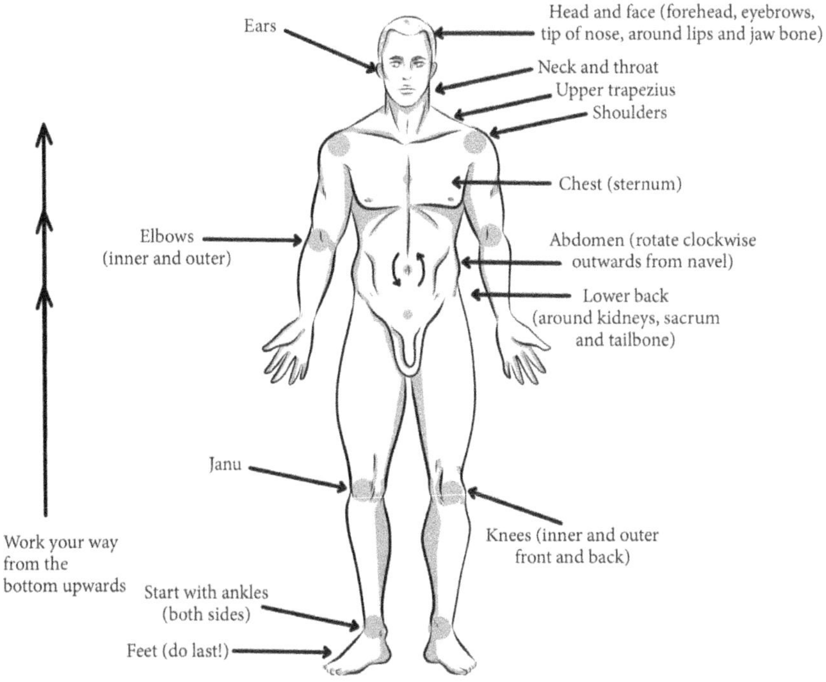

Figure 9.2: Daily Oil Massage Sequence

The most common base oil used for massage in Āyurveda is sesame oil. It is considered to be one of the best oils for mitigating vāta because it is warming and nourishing. Herbal massage oils also use sesame oil, and the infused herb will depend on the condition it is intended to treat. The best oil to use for muscular pain is Mahānārāyaṇa Oil, which contains guggul, a painkilling resin that is used very effectively in Āyurveda. This oil is quite easy to get hold of online and it is worth using as part of a bigger pain-management programme.

In the UK, other base oils are popular, such as sweet almond. This is also a nice oil with vāta-pacifying properties.

5. BATHING AND SUDATION

Once you have applied oil to your body, you are ready to bathe. If your routine is focused on managing vāta doṣa, it is best to soak in a warm bath but not for more than about 15–20 minutes. Any longer and the water will sap your energy and you will feel tired for the rest of the day. Oil and heat are the two key methods used in Āyurveda to minimize the negative effects of vāta, so if you are heading towards the age of vāta (60 plus) then take these points seriously.

A younger person will enjoy a quick shower, but be careful not to use too much soap, which can dry out the skin and alkalize the important acid mantle of the skin, which is generally between 4.5 and 6.2 on the pH scale. It is best to use soap on the sweaty bits only. Some people like to use Āyurvedic soap, which is soap with some Āyurvedic herbs added. It is important to note that soap is soap; there isn't much added therapeutic value in using a scented or herbal soap.

SOAP NUTS (SAPINDUS)

If you really want to go to town on natural products, you can try soap nuts or soap berries.

They are quite easy to get hold of and can actually be used for a wide variety of cleaning needs, including yourself. They are certainly worth trying if you have very sensitive skin that reacts badly to petroleum-based products.

SUDATION (SVEDANA)

From an Āyurvedic perspective, one of the goals of using heat therapeutically is to make you sweat a little. Heat in itself is vāta and kapha pacifying, but when it induces a mild sweat, it is even better because it opens the pores and releases some toxins too. In Āyurvedic clinics, you are usually put into a steam box for a few minutes after receiving an oil massage. The therapist waits for a mild sweat to appear on your forehead and then takes you out to bathe. Obviously, most of us won't have the luxury of a steam box at home, but infrared saunas are now becoming more affordable so it wouldn't be out of the question. They are safe when used sensibly and don't take up too much space. Put it on your wish list. You never know!

6. MOUTH ABLUTIONS (TEETH, GARGLING, TONGUE)

Here is another interesting technique that we overlook in the west: the art of swilling and oil pulling.

OIL PULLING (GAṆḌŪṢA)

The art of swilling oil around your mouth and gargling is known as Gaṇḍūṣa. The ancient Āyurvedic texts make all sorts of claims about its benefits, such as its ability to detoxify and purify the body, etc., but let's be sensible. Sesame oil – medicated or otherwise – will certainly help with oral health. The salivary glands will be stimulated and send signals to your gut to fire up the agni in anticipation of breakfast. As with many claims made in the yoga texts, whenever any technique is believed to stimulate agni, this makes way for all manner of possibilities, but this is more to do with literary style than observable fact.

If you have time, dedicate five minutes of your bathroom routine to oil pulling. You will certainly notice improvements in oral health and hygiene, and any other benefits would be a bonus. Some books tell you to do it for 15 minutes. This is not realistic from my experience, unless you have lots of time to kill. Even five minutes is difficult for the average working person, but that's a good time to aim for.

7. NOSE (JALA NETI/NASYA)[3]

Nasal irrigation is one of the many ancient Āyurvedic techniques described in the *HYP* that has been adopted in modern yoga practice. It has proven to be so useful that it is even used in the UK National Health Service. It is very simple to do once you have got the hang of it. The idea is to slowly pour salty water in through one nostril and pass it out of the other. The saline solution bathes the nasal cavity and passes out of the other nostril because of the angle of the head. Once you have mastered the technique and understand the pitfalls, you can teach it to your own students. It is a great way of clearing excess mucus out of the sinuses and improving mental clarity (see Appendix 5).

8. YOGA PRACTICE (ĀSANA, PRĀṆĀYĀMA)

Your daily yoga practice should be a simple sequence that includes all the key posture groups. The dynamism of the sequence will depend on the experience, personality and goals of you or your students; however, in general, there should be:

1. A warm-up sequence that involves joint mobility.
2. A gentle dynamic sequence that coordinates breath with movement and raises the heart rate a little.
3. Back bends.
4. Forward bends.
5. Twists.
6. A short relaxation followed by a breathing practice.

3 National Centre for Biotechnology Information (2009). *Saline Nasal Irrigation for Upper Respiratory Conditions.* Accessed on 24/2/2021 at www.ncbi.nlm.nih.gov/pmc/articles/PMC2778074.

9. BREAKFAST

In Āyurveda, they say that you should have breakfast like a princess, lunch like a queen and dinner like a pauper. If you are heavily influenced by kapha doṣa, it is best to limit yourself to two meals a day, which means you may want to miss breakfast, as long as you are not compensating by gorging in the evening. If you find this happening, train yourself to have breakfast to help balance your blood sugars more evenly throughout the day.

What you prefer to eat for breakfast is largely cultural, but whatever it is, make sure it is wholesome food that isn't mouldy or over-processed. Be careful of food combining, especially if your digestion is showing signs of weariness. Fruit and yoghurt do not combine well according to Āyurveda and neither do fish and dairy.

Daytime: work and community

We all need to be busy doing work we consider to be of value to ourselves and ideally to others too. The nature of what we do depends largely on our prakṛti. Dharma means 'duty'; our first duty is to the wellbeing of our community and our next is to our own wellbeing (see 'Prakṛti and Dharma' in Chapter 3 for more on Dharma).

Evening

10. PRACTISE YOGA NIDRĀ BETWEEN 4PM AND 6PM

Yoga Nidrā, as taught by the Bihar School of Yoga,[4] is one of the most effective practices for balancing vāta doṣa. It is best, though not essential, to practise it between 4pm and 6pm because vāta is dominant at this time so the benefits will be felt more greatly (see Chapter 11).

4 Bihar School of Yoga (2020). *Homepage*. Accessed on 24/2/2021 at www.biharyoga.net.

11. MEDITATE AT DUSK (20 MINUTES)

Vāta controls all the sandhyās or junctions so dusk is a good time to meditate. In the yoga scriptures there are lots of dos and don'ts for this auspicious time. It is thought that the solar and lunar energies (ida and piṅgala) are in balance at dawn and dusk so there is less mental turbulence. Many traditions encourage two sittings a day of at least 20 minutes.

12. EVENING MEAL BETWEEN 6PM AND 8PM

It is important not to eat too late. It takes about four hours for your stomach to process a large meal before it passes into the small intestine, so try to have your main meal by 7pm so that the food doesn't have to sit in your stomach when you go to bed. The evening meal is tricky because, on the one hand, Āyurveda says that it should be the lightest meal of the day, but on the other hand, many families get together round the dinner table in the evening and use it for social bonding. I don't have any answers to this unfortunately, as it is a cultural issue. I will say, however, that if you are experiencing digestive problems, you will need to adhere to Āyurvedic recommendations more strictly.

13. COMMUNITY ACTIVITY AND ENJOYMENT

It's important to build some fun into your day. Time with your friends, family, loved ones or even on your own. Time to let your hair down, laugh and enjoy yourself. In Āyurveda, sukha, or enjoyment, is an important goal to recognize. Sukha (pleasure) and duḥkha (pain or suffering) are inspired by yoga but in this context refer to Kāma, one of the four goals of life. Kāma means 'desire'. It is important to know what we want, because what we think we want becomes a focal point and key source of pleasure. Most of us have everything we need to be joyful right now, so make time to celebrate.

14. OLEATION

Light oleation before bed is useful for pacifying vāta if you have had a busy day. Just a light oiling of your feet; and if you have been on your feet all day, you may want to do your knees and sacrum too. A thin film of oil is enough, otherwise it will stain your sheets. You may prefer to follow it with a warm bath so that you are properly relaxed before going to bed.

15. QUIET MEDITATION

In the evening or before bed, try to leave a good 20 minutes for quiet sitting. It will calm the mind and prepare you well for sleep. You will enjoy better-quality rest and even dream more sweetly.

16. BEDTIME: NO LATER THAN 11PM

It is important not to go to bed too late. Pitta doṣa is dominant between 10pm and 2am, so if you stay up too long, you will get hungry again. The idea is to be asleep by the time pitta reaches its peak so that your body can get on with properly digesting food and replenishing your tissues. If you get insomnia during pitta time, it could be a sign that pitta doṣa is aggravated, especially if it is accompanied by other pitta symptoms like heat, acidity or hunger.

Seasonal regimens (Ṛtucharyā)

The word 'Ṛtucharyā' literally means 'discipline or regimen [charya] of the season [ritu]' and goes hand in hand with dinacaryā. It is another example of how Āyurveda acknowledges the importance of time and how life operates through cyclic relationships between the sun, moon and earth. Charaka highlights the importance of the impact of the solar and lunar energy on life on earth.

In the northern hemisphere, between 21 December (winter solstice) and 21 June (summer solstice) the sun gradually increases in power. It dries out the environment and uses up the rasa, or life sap, therein.

From 21 June onwards, the sun gradually begins to weaken again, and the moon builds its strength until it reaches the culmination of its power by 21 December. As it gains strength, it is able to replenish the earth with rasa.

This vital relationship forms the basis of the influence of the weather on the gunas or qualities in the environment. It is important for us to understand our relationship with the seasons. We may notice that over time, this relationship changes. We may once have been sun worshippers but now find that too much heat and light aggravate us.

As we move into the age of vāta (after 60 for most people) we experience more dryness. Our ojas has reduced and we no longer have the strength and vitality of our youth. The nurturing energy of the moon may become more important to us or vice versa. We may find that we actually depend more on the energy of sunlight. We may crave warmer climes to mitigate the drying effects of vāta doṣa.

Take this quick test and see how it is for you.

TABLE 9.1: SEASONAL PREFERENCES

1	Which season do you like the most? Is there a link with the environment?
2	Which season do you like the least? What effect does it have?
3	On a scale of 1–10, how much impact do the weather patterns have on your sense of wellness (1 being not a problem at all and 10 being very problematic)? You may want to write a few words to help you understand yourself better.
	Heat
	Cold
	Wind
	Rain
	Snow
	Cloudy
	Dry
	Humid
	Darkness

Self-care and yoga teaching through the seasons

There are actually six seasons in India because monsoon is a season in itself; but in the west, we work with four seasons. It is more useful to think in terms of our relationship with weather fluctuations and light than to generalize.

SPRING

The spring equinox marks the beginning of spring and in the UK continues till the summer solstice on 21 June, which marks the beginning of summer. The first degree of Aries is marked by 21 March, so nature is flush with burgeoning creative energy. It is time to clear out the cobwebs of winter, both internally and externally.

In the beginning of spring, accumulated kapha doṣa begins to melt and liquify due to the warmer weather. This can lead to all sorts of respiratory disorders as the body attempts to expel the liquified doṣa. It is best to avoid kapha-aggravating foods at this time. That is, foods that are heavy, sour, sweet and fatty.

Sleeping during the day is something Āyurveda generally frowns upon because it affects the strength of our agni, so this should be particularly avoided in this season when kapha is high.

If the weather is still cool, heat can be increased to help mobilize the body and clear excess phlegm; but as the weather warms up, warming regimens should be reduced.

Early spring is also a good time for fasting. Take ten days out to do a gentle fast. There are many ways of doing this, but the best method is a juice fast. It is not as stressful as a water fast and you are able to retain all your electrolytes with vegetable juices like carrot and celery.

As the weather warms up, pitta will start to accrue, so start planning your salads and cooling foods ready for the summer.

It is also worth pointing out that the spring is the season of love. The birds and the bees, so to speak, so it is a good time to organize a romantic getaway with your beloved or arrange some dates!

YOGA TEACHING IN THE SPRING

For general classes, dynamic practices should be increased at this time. Classes should include more vinyasas, Sūrya Namaskaras (Sun Salutations), agni-kindling practices, Kapālabhātī, Bhastrikā, Sūrya Bheda and pair work.

SUMMER

Summer in the UK is from 21 June to 20 September (the day before the autumn equinox). The solar energy peaks at the beginning of summer and begins its descent even though we may not necessarily feel its full intensity till July. The heat has dried out the earth so vāta and pitta will naturally increase. We can eat more raw foods like salads at this time and enjoy sweet fruits. We should avoid foods that will increase heat and dryness further, that is sour, salty and spicy foods. We should spend more time in a cool natural environment like a forest or green countryside. It is also useful to wear cooling gems like pearls.

PITTA CLEANSING

At the end of the summer, perhaps late August or early September, pitta doṣa will be high, so it is actually a good time to do a pitta cleanse. For ten days, take two to three capsules of Triphala every night an hour before bed. Triphala is popular formulation used in Āyurveda that will act as a mild purgative when taken in this way, so you will be purging the excess pitta from the digestive tract over a period of time. Other methods are to drink dandelion coffee, which is really dandelion root. The bitter taste will help to cleanse the liver. It is also a good diuretic so it will flush out the kidneys too. If you are not well enough to use purgatives, taking aloe vera juice will help to pacify pitta doṣa; but if possible, it is much better to explore ways of purging in some way. Get advice from your local Āyurvedic practitioner.

YOGA TEACHING IN THE SUMMER

It is tempting to practise more vigorously in the summer because we generally feel lighter, but we have to be mindful of burning ourselves out and weakening further. Mild sweating can be a good way of excreting bodily acids, but generating too much heat will not serve us well in the long run. We need to retain our fluid levels by making sure we are well hydrated and focus more on cooling yoga practices that include twists, forward bends, meditation, Sitāli and Seetkari prāṇāyāma and devotional practices.

AUTUMN

Autumn in the UK is between 21 September and 20 December. Autumn is a dry season so vāta will begin to accumulate. As we progress towards December, the weather will get colder and windier, so we have to start looking after vāta doṣa again. No more cold, raw foods. It is time to reintroduce nourishing soups, hot casseroles and sweet, oily foods.

YOGA TEACHING IN THE AUTUMN

Pay attention to the changing weather. If it is getting cold and windy, vāta is your main consideration. If it is getting cold and wet, both vāta and kapha need to be managed. Vāta is always the main priority because it is the master doṣa.

People like to get back into routines in September (Virgo season), so consider teaching a fixed sequence that students can practise at home. Create a handout with stick men for a class of no more than 30–40 minutes and email it to them. Include all the key posture groups (standing, sitting, back bends, forward bends, twists and inversions) so that your students can bring vāta back into balance. When you are teaching live, vary the pace and rhythm of the sequence with different themes (see Chapter 10).

WINTER

Winter in the UK is from 21 December to 20 March. The lunar energy peaks at the start of the winter so we have a lot of latent energy to burn off. Unlike the daily cycle, where agni or digestive power is strongest at midday, in the annual cycle, agni is actually stronger in the winter because it has to be. The lunar environment imposes itself and forces the body to galvanize itself to maintain its integrity. Your appetite is therefore likely to be stronger in the winter, and it is normal to want to eat more stodgy foods. Vāta will be increasing from the cold, and kapha will be increasing from the dampness, but pitta will be in balance. You will be able to enjoy saunas and warm oil massages to help your circulation.

YOGA TEACHING IN THE WINTER

This is the season when stronger dynamic practices will be helpful for an average general class. They will help to maintain the strength of the agni, improve overall body heat and circulation and mitigate the heaviness of the dark wintery environment.

You can teach dynamically at this time. Students will feel great and there will not be any deleterious effects. It is always important to assess the needs of your group, however. I find that I can enjoy yoga more in a heated studio in the winter, but this is not so in the summer. The idea of heat helping to lubricate the joints so you can stretch further and improve your range of movement comes into its own during this season.

Teaching in the four seasons

SPRING (21 MARCH TO 20 JUNE)

- Dynamic and lightening practices (laṅghana) to clear winter kapha and take advantage of spring energy.
- Avoid heavy, fatty foods. Have light, warm and fresh food. Use warming spices like ginger, cinnamon, cardamon, turmeric and black pepper.
- This is a good season for strong exercise and intermittent fasting or juice fasting for short periods.

SUMMER (21 JUNE TO 20 SEPTEMBER)

- Cooling practices.
- Meditation.
- Prāṇāyāma.
- Outdoor living.
- Sunbathing till 11am or after 4pm.

- Use cooling foods and herbs like aloe vera, coconut, watermelon, peaches, dates and other sweet fruits.
- Salads that include fresh fennel can also be enjoyed in this season if agni is normal.

AUTUMN (21 SEPTEMBER TO 20 DECEMBER)

- Pitta- and vāta-pacifying practices.
- Restorative practices.
- Joint mobility.
- Gentle dynamic, repetitive sequences.
- Keep the mind stable with simple routine āsana with ujjayi breath and simple daily prāṇāyāma.
- Early autumn is good for clearing excess pitta doṣa by eating lots of steamed fresh green vegetables like broccoli, kale and cauliflower. Fenugreek, ginger, dandelion root, fennel, coriander and parsley are good for this season.

WINTER (21 DECEMBER TO 20 MARCH)

- Gentle, warming practices.
- Kapālabhātī.
- Bhastrikā.
- Sūrya Namaskara (Sun Salutation).
- Sūrya Bheda.
- Keep the body warm and the mind active during the winter.
- Remain as active as possible but avoid overexposure to strong wind, damp and cold.

- This is a good time to eat heavier foods, because agni is strong in the winter. It is a good time to replenish ojas in preparation for the new season.
- No detox programmes should be carried out if the weather is cold.

Your morning regimen

TABLE 9.2: YOUR DAILY REGIMEN

	Activity	Yes	No
1.	Wake up between 5am and 7am, ideally before or around sunrise.		
2	Chant your favourite mantra 11 times within the first hour of waking.		
3	Empty your bowels and bladder.		
4	Brush your skin all over, using a natural bristle brush. (This is best for kapha types; miss it out if you have dry skin.)		
5	Apply sesame oil to the body (miss this out if you have oily skin) and leave it on until you bathe.		
6	Brush your teeth (using herbal powder if you have some).		
7	Scrape your tongue.		
6	Oil pull for one minute with a teaspoon of sesame oil (Gaṇḍūṣa).		
7	Have a warm shower or bath, depending on the time of year and your constitution (too much heat is not good for excess pitta). Wash off most of the sesame oil using Āyurvedic soap but don't overdo it.		
8	Practise jala neti (nasal cleansing using a neti pot) if you have been properly taught. This is best for those who have a lot of mucus. Avoid this if you have high vāta or high blood pressure (see Appendix 5).		
9	After drying, reapply a little sesame or coconut oil to the feet, ears and head, and massage well. If you get back pain, rub a little into your sacrum as well.		
10	Drink a glass of warm water with a squeeze of lemon.		
11	Practise some gentle āsana to warm up the spine and hips.		
12	Practise gentle prāṇāyāma to nourish your prāṇic body.		
13	Get dressed, using colours that will enhance your mood.		
14	Have a good breakfast.		
15	Remain mindful of your day's activities and remember to smile and be kind!		

Keeping an Āyurvedic diary

There is no better way to get to know yourself than to keep an Āyurvedic diary. How does this differ from a normal diary? An Āyurvedic diary helps you to identify your strengths and weaknesses from an Āyurvedic perspective. Once you have got the hang of it, you can share this idea with your students.

You can organize your diary in any way you like. From my experience, it is best not to have too many categories to think about, because you can get tired of it and it can become meaningless.

A meaningful diary is one that:

- Provides a proper platform for self-reflection rather than box ticking.
- Can potentially provide data as evidence of bad or good habits you may have. Many of us are in denial about our bad habits, but when we see them written in black and white, we cannot deny the truth of our behaviour.
- You enjoy engaging with most of the time. The self-reflective journey does not appeal to all personality types so if you prefer to collect data then you may prefer a tick-box type of template where you are recording what you ate, how long you practised yoga, what poses you did and so on.
- Should relate to your goal-setting programme. If it doesn't, then revisit your goals and see if they need to be amended or made more relevant.

Here is a universal format you can adapt to suit yourself.

TABLE 9.4: ĀYURVEDIC DIARY TEMPLATE

Name:		Date:	Time:
What three things did you want to achieve today and how successful were you?			
Yoga: What practices did you do today and for how long?	Āsana:	Prāṇāyāma:	Mantra:
	Seva (service in community):	Bhakti (devotional practices):	Jnana (study of scriptures):
Diet: What did you eat today?	Number of fruits:	Number of vegetables:	Grains:
	Animal proteins:	Dairy:	Processed:
Activities	Work time:	Leisure time:	Creative time:
	Exercise:	Family/community time:	Quiet time:
Notes (any key words, things to remember, things to change, strategies)			

—Chapter 10—

COURSE AND LESSON PLANNING WITH ĀYURVEDIC THEMES

Teaching with an Āyurvedic focus can enrich your classes and courses enormously because your classes are more likely to hit the mark and meet the needs of your students.

In this chapter, we will take a closer look at how to build a course plan with an Āyurvedic theme and then create a few lesson plans that can be used again and again.

Course planning

What is a course plan?

A course plan is a programme of study or practice that leads towards the achievement of a goal. The goal usually includes a set of skills and underpinning knowledge that enables you to do something competently. The number of hours a course covers is the time needed to build up the knowledge and develop the skills to achieve the overall aim. The skills and knowledge learned are usually progressive and cumulative.

Aims and learning outcomes

The overall aims of the course need to be established at the outset, followed by a breakdown of everything students have to learn in order to achieve them. The aim of a course may be set by you, the tutor, or an outside body that sets the standards. The learning outcomes relate to what the students need to learn in the process.

Here is a useful template for creating a course plan.

TABLE 10.1: COURSE PLAN TEMPLATE

Course title:		
Start date:	End date:	Duration/total hours:
Format (e.g., one 90-minute class per week for 10 weeks):		
Location (if known):		
Level of group:		
Rationale for the programme (What is your vision and how do you envisage its delivery?):		
Overall aim (What are your key goals for the programme?):		
Learning outcomes (By the end of the programme, students should be able to...): 1. 2. 3.		

Teaching methods:

Day	Theme	Aims (To enable/ familiarize students to/with...):	Learning outcomes (By the end of each session, students should be able to...):
1			
2			
3			
4			

How to build a yoga course plan with an Āyurvedic theme

How do you teach yoga with an Āyurvedic approach? We have reached the crux of the matter so now we need to consider what is achievable and appropriate for our students.

We may have spent a lot of time studying the fundamental principles of Āyurveda, learning about the doṣas, elements, dhātus, marma points and so on, but sharing any of this knowledge with our yoga students is hugely challenging. Students may not have even heard of Āyurveda, so how do you keep them motivated without having to give long lectures, and how do you keep it simple without losing the essence of what Āyurveda is about? Striking a balance is very tricky.

Here is the kind of course I think you should teach. I have used the template above with all the sections filled in. You can obviously tweak the course in any way you want to suit your students.

TABLE 10.2: COURSE PLAN SAMPLE

Course title: Yoga with an Āyurvedic approach

Start date: **End date:** **Duration/total hours:** 15 hours

Format (e.g., one 90-minute class per week for 10 weeks): One 90-minute class for 10 weeks

Location (if known):

Rationale for the programme (What is your vision and how do you envisage its delivery?):

Students can enrich their yoga practice by taking personal and environmental factors into consideration. These factors can be assessed from an Āyurvedic perspective and can help them decide how they can adapt their practice according to the time of the year, the time of the day, the seasons, the weather and their own personal needs. By teaching them about the five elements, three doṣas, three yogic gunas (sattva, rajas and tamas) and the 20 gunas, they will be able to adapt their own practice accordingly. Outside this remit, I will limit the course to some key ideas pertaining to the importance of daily routines.

Overall aim (What are your key goals for the programme?):

To familiarize students with the basic principles of Āyurveda and enable them to assess their home yoga practice and make adjustments accordingly.

Learning outcomes (By the end of the programme, students should be able to...):

1. Differentiate between the five elements (earth, water, fire, air and space).
2. Differentiate between the three doṣas (vāta, pitta and kapha) and articulate their own relationship with them.
3. Describe the effects of the doṣas using the Āyurvedic gunas (qualities).
4. Relate their own mental and emotional states to the three yogic gunas (sattva, rajas and tamas).
5. Adapt their āsana practice according to their experience of the gunas as expressed by the three doṣas.
6. Explain the importance of establishing a good daily routine based on Āyurvedic principles.

Teaching methods:

Each week, there will be an Āyurvedic theme that is supported by a handout. The theme will be briefly introduced at the beginning of the class (5 minutes), and about 10 minutes will be allowed at the end of the class to feedback on their understanding and relevance to the day's practice.

Āsana work will be group led and there may be some pair work to help raise awareness.

There will be a handout that provides key information before each session that students will be expected to read.

Students will be split into small groups at the end of each session to discuss their understanding and whether their learning outcomes have been met for that session.

They will have about 5 minutes for this before the final plenary and feedback (10 minutes).

Total discussion time: 20 minutes (5 minutes at the start, 5 minutes of group discussion, 10 minutes of group feedback).

Total āsana practice time: 60 minutes per session.

Total breathing and meditation time: 10 minutes per session.

Day	Theme	Aims (To enable/ familiarize students to/with...):	Learning outcomes (By the end of each session, students should be able to...):
1	Introducing the Āyurvedic gunas in yoga practice. Introducing the idea of giving to the ground and finding support from the ground.	To familiarize students with the experience of their bodies and minds using some key Āyurvedic guna polarities and how they relate to the ground.	Assess their own bodies and minds in general āsana and breathing practice on the experiential scale of: • hot and cold • heavy and light • still and moving • rough and smooth • sharp and soft • even and irregular • solid and spacious. Describe their experience of giving and receiving from the ground.
2	Working with earth and water.	To familiarize students with the qualities of earth and water and relate them to the body/mind experience.	Apply the techniques of visualization and body sensation to the metaphysical concepts of earth and water. Discuss the key functions of kapha doṣa.
3	Working with air and space.	To familiarize students with the qualities of air and space and relate them to the body/mind experience.	Apply the techniques of visualization and body sensation to the metaphysical concepts of air and space. Discuss the key functions of vāta doṣa.
4	Working with fire and water.	To familiarize students with the qualities of fire and water and relate them to the body/mind experience.	Apply the techniques of visualization and body sensation to the metaphysical concepts of fire and water. Discuss the key functions of pitta doṣa.
5	A closer look at vāta.	To explore vāta doṣa more deeply in relation to āsana and breathing practice. To introduce the importance of daily routines.	Apply the techniques of visualization and body sensation to the movement of vāta around the body. Name key postures that help to open the front hips. Practise joint mobility with breath coordination. Observe the behaviour of their breath in a seated and lying position. Discuss appropriate times for vāta-harmonizing practice.

Day	Theme	Aims (To enable/ familiarize students to/with…):	Learning outcomes (By the end of each session, students should be able to…):
6	A closer look at pitta.	To explore pitta doṣa more deeply in āsana and breathing practice.	Apply the techniques of visualization and body sensation to the quality of movement and seats of pitta doṣa. Name key postures that help to stretch and tone the abdomen Practise cooling and surrendering practices using the breath and mind. Discuss appropriate times for pitta-harmonizing practice.
7	A closer look at kapha.	To explore kapha doṣa more deeply in āsana and breathing practice.	Apply the techniques of visualization and body sensation to the quality and pace of movement. Name key postures that help to open the chest and raise the heart rate. Practise warming and mobilizing practices that build up incrementally. Discuss appropriate times for kapha-harmonizing practice.
8	Working more closely with the breath.	To explore different ways of using the breath in yoga practice and how it impacts on the doṣas. To revise the influence of doṣas on daily cycles.	Practise āsana for prāṇāyāma preparation. Practise an appropriate variation of: • Kapālabhātī • Nādi Śodhana • Sitāli • Seetkari.
9	Putting it all together 1.	To enable students to integrate their learning by creating their own 10-minute sequence in groups.	Assess the current environment and suggest an appropriate sequence, theme and focus for the practice. The practice will consider: • environmental gunas • time of the day • time of the year • time of the week.

10	Putting it all together 2.	To create a platform for students to share their learning and experience with their peers.	Assess the current environment and suggest two different sequences based on different themes related to: • environmental gunas • time of the day • time of the year • time of the week. Assess their overall understanding of the Āyurvedic approach and share their experience

Lesson planning

Once you have created the broad strokes of your course plan, you need to consider the detail of how you will deliver your course. This detailed outline of exactly what you will be teaching is called a lesson plan and in many ways is a smaller version of the same format.

Proper lesson planning will involve a minute-by-minute consideration of exactly what will be taught, in what order and how long each activity will take. It is the bread and butter of good quality teaching and a necessary rite of passage, however tedious it may be. Lesson planning gets quicker and you will eventually be able to rustle one up in your head in a matter of minutes, but until that point is reached, properly planned classes are better in every way. I have sometimes heard teachers say that they never use a lesson plan, but this is usually because they are very experienced and are able to build an element of spontaneity into a class without losing its balance and integrity.

Here is a sample of what your lesson plan might look like from day 1 of your course plan.

TABLE 10.3: LESSON PLAN SAMPLE

Āyurvedic theme: Introducing the Āyurvedic and Yogic Gunas	**Date:** **Time:**

Aim: To familiarize students with the experience of their bodies and mind using some key Āyurvedic guna polarities and how they relate to the ground.
To explore the idea of giving to the ground and finding support from the ground.

Learning outcomes (By the end of the programme, students should be able to…):

1. Assess their own bodies and minds in general āsana and breathing practice on the experiential scale of:
    - hot and cold
    - heavy and light
    - still and moving
    - rough and smooth
    - sharp and soft
    - even and irregular
    - solid and spacious.
2. Describe the experience of giving to and finding support from the ground.

Time	**Activity**	**Purpose/rationale**	**Modifications/ precautions**
00–10	Introduce the concept of gunas/qualities and how we experience them in our bodies and environment.	To establish the working theme for the practice.	Make sure students with special considerations are sitting near the front.
10–15	Breath and body awareness in Savasana (Corpse pose). Exploring: • heavy and light • smooth breathing • even breathing • starting quality of mind • becoming aware of how much we can give to the ground.	To connect with the contrasting qualities in a relaxed pose.	Support for back, knees and neck as appropriate.
15–25	Warm-up sequence in supine position • Ankle rotations • Sucirandhrasana (Eye of Needle pose) • Setu Bandhasana (Bridge pose) • Ananda Balasana (Happy Baby) • Back rolls	To warm up the body and mobilize the joints.	Caution against torqueing in the knees, lower back and sacral compression.

25–35	Sūrya Namaskara (Sun Salutation): 6 times. Exploring: • stillness and movement • hot and cold sensations • even and uneven breathing.	To connect with the contrasting qualities in a dynamic sequence.	
35–50	Standing poses • Vīrabhadrāsana 2 (Warrior 2) • Utthita Pārśvakoṇāsana (Extended Side Angle pose) • Trikoṇāsana (Triangle pose) • Forward bends • Vṛkṣāsana (Tree pose) Exploring the qualities of: • stable and light • sharp and soft focus • heating yet grounding • stillness and movement • giving to the ground.	To connect with contrasting qualities in standing poses. To raise kinaesthetic awareness of how to relate to the ground in āsana practice.	Ensure that there is minimal compression on the cervical and lumbar spine. Ensure that the knees do not bear unnecessary and excessive load. Check that the rise in heart rate does not cause dizziness or light-headedness.
50–60	Back bends • Urdhva Mukha Śvānāsana (Upward Facing Dog) • Bhujaṅgāsana (Cobra pose) • Dhanurasana (Bow pose) Exploring the qualities of: • sharp and soft focus • how to give to the ground and find support from it in back bends.	To connect with contrasting qualities in prone back bends. To experiment with giving and receiving in back bends.	Caution against sustained or excessive lower back and cervical compression.
60–65	Seated twist • Ardhā Matsyendrāsana (Half Spinal Twist) Exploring the qualities of: • light and heavy • solid and spacious.	To connect with contrasting qualities in a seated twist. How to use the ground to create more lightness.	Caution against excessive rotation in the sacroiliac and cervical spine.

Time	Activity	Purpose/rationale	Modifications/ precautions
65–70	Seated forward bend • Paścimottānāsana (Seated Forward Bend) Exploring: • heavy and light sensations through giving to and receiving from the ground • sharp and soft focus • even breathing.	To connect with contrasting qualities in a seated forward bend.	Cautious of anterior compression in the lumbar and sacrum in particular but also in the spine as a whole.
70–80	Final relaxation • Revisiting the contrasting qualities	To relax the body, integrate and consolidate experience.	Ensure that the body is comfortable, warm and supported.
80–90	Feedback on student experience. Q&A.	To consolidate cognitive and affective learning.	

Here is a blank template for your own lesson plans.

TABLE 10.4: LESSON PLAN TEMPLATE

Āyurvedic theme:	Date: Time:
Aims:	
Learning outcomes:	

Time	Activity	Purpose/ rationale	Modifications/ precautions	Notes

How to build a lesson plan

Pick a theme and develop an aim. If you are an experienced teacher, here are some themes you can pick out of a hat and teach.

TABLE 10.5: LESSON PLANNING THEMES

Theme	Aim
Animals that express doshic archetypes	To explore the imagined qualities of some common animals in āsana practice such as the slug (kapha), tiger (pitta), bird (vāta) and elephant (kapha).
Working with space	To explore space within and around the body in āsana practice (vāta).
Working with rhythm	To engage with slower and faster rhythm in movement and how to synchronize with breath.
Joint freedom	To harmonize vāta doṣa by mobilizing the knees, shoulders, hips and spine.
Cooling	To cool down the body and mind using twists, forward bends and cooling techniques (pitta pacifying).
Revitalizing agni	To stimulate the agni or metabolic power of the body with heating āsana and prāṇāyāma practices (agni stimulating).
Nourishing	To cultivate a sense of self-care and nourishment through static āsana work, visualization and relaxation (Rasāyana: rejuvenation).
Laṅghana (lightening)	To cultivate lightness of being by working with standing poses, back bends and visualization.
Rooting	To raise awareness of how we connect with the ground by rooting through the hands and feet (vāta/kapha: working with gravity).
Dṛṣṭis (focused gazing)	To cultivate ekagrata (one-pointedness) through āsana and meditation practice (raising sattva guna and mental sharpness: pitta).
Astrological symbolism (Prakṛti)	To experiment with astrological symbolism in āsana, visualization and meditation practice (tridoshic).
Senses	To engage the senses in āsana, prāṇāyāma and meditation practice.
Meditation on the prāṇic body	To cultivate awareness of pranaymayakosha or the pranic body in asana, pranayama and meditation.

There is obviously a lot of scope here so don't try and teach any of the above until you have read the whole book and understood the context of how to work with these themes. Many of the themes are explored in subsequent chapters.

ANIMALS THAT EXPRESS DOSHIC ARCHETYPES

When we are learning about the Āyurvedic gunas, it is useful to think of animals that express those qualities so we can get a better feel for them. From our point of view, elephants are relatively large, solid, calm and graceful animals. We could therefore associate elephants with the key characteristics of kapha doṣa. Birds are relatively light, quick and mobile so we could associate them with vāta doṣa. Tigers have sharp teeth and use aggression to be able to meet their dietary needs; this behaviour could be associated with pitta doṣa. The next time you observe nature, notice the different qualities that animals and indeed plants imbibe and express. An owl is heavier and larger than a robin, so it has more kapha qualities. A hamster is quick, but a mouse is quicker (vāta) and a rat is more aggressive (pitta).

All living things express the five elements to varying degrees, and their interaction is relative. We make comparisons on the basis of our own perception. There is nothing objective beyond the relative. Everything lives on a spectrum of self-expression. Using animals when teaching āsana is a good way of conveying this. Many āsanas have animal names, so you might want to pinpoint and highlight certain qualities associated with such animals. Here are some examples.

TABLE 10.6: ANIMALS AND ĀSANA

Animal and āsana	Some suggested qualities
Cat pose	Playful and agile.
Crocodile pose	Relaxed yet powerful. Draws strength from the earth.
Crow pose	Light yet steady.
Downward Facing Dog pose	Reverential yet playful.
Eagle pose	Bound and safe. Delicate balance.
Fish pose	Open but awkward. Trusting.
Horse pose	Strong and steady.
Pigeon pose	Long, open and light.
Snake pose	Strong yet supported as one lifts away from the ground.
Tiger pose	Sharp and predatory.

WORKING WITH SPACE

We are used to identifying with our body as a tangible object that we can see, feel, smell and touch. But let us not forget that the way our body is arranged is equally dependent on how it utilizes space. Any structure needs space to inhabit. It seems like a bizarre notion because we take space for granted, but Āyurveda reminds us that space is alive too and our relationship with it can vary. Consider a situation where you didn't have enough space to live, breathe and express yourself. Some people hate enclosed spaces, and others feel uncomfortable in open spaces.

Our sense of space informs our sense of place. In other words, we have a sense of what we need to feel comfortable and supported. Exploring space in āsana practice is quite fascinating. We can consider the existing spaces inside us that we take for granted, like inside our nose, mouth, sinuses and chest. We can also consider the space around our bodies and how close we allow people to get to us before we feel like our space has been invaded. It is also interesting to explore the space created via the different shapes we create through āsana practice. The space between the legs and the floor in Trikoṇāsana (Triangle pose) for example, or the space between the fingers and hands in Vīrabhadrāsana 1 (Warrior 1), or the space between the hands and the floor in Adho Mukha Svanāsana (Downward Facing Dog pose). It is a really interesting proprioceptive experience.

WORKING WITH RHYTHM

This seems like an odd idea because rhythm tends to make us think of music and dance. However, there is an intrinsic relationship between rhythms and cycles. Our heart beats to a rhythm. We breath rhythmically and even our gait has a rhythmic pattern that can be measured. Āsana practice helps raise our awareness of bodily rhythms and we can learn to observe them.

It is best not to interfere with natural breathing until you have gained some mastery over the body; and it is certainly not advised if you have any health issues, particularly vāta-related ones.

Prāṇāyāma is one way of working with breathing patterns. We learn to control the length of the inhalation and exhalation, as well as how long we should retain the breath. Retaining the breath for different ratios of time affects us in slightly different ways.

Synchronization between breath and movement

In dynamic yoga practice, we synchronize body movement with our breathing. We usually raise our arms on an inhalation, for example, and lower on an exhalation. In some traditions of āsana, sequences can be created using this basic breath/movement relationship. When we move in time with other students, it often feels effortless because we feel as though we are being carried by the synchronized rhythm of the group as a whole.

Meditating on rhythms

There are other ways of using this idea. Have you ever tried to feel your own pulse between your eyebrows? It takes a lot of practice but is eminently possible and quite mesmerizing. How about observing the rhythmic movement of your diaphragm? What usually happens below your radar is now happening within your radar. The next time you go for a walk, try synchronizing your gait with your breath. It's an ideal way of practising walking meditation. If you have a mantra, you can attach the mantra to the breath too.

JOINT FREEDOM

The notion of freeing joints is a bit misleading because in order to free joints, we have to free up the tensions in the tissues that connect to them. Very bendy people usually have naturally loose ligaments which, by the way, is not necessarily a good thing. Hyper-flexibility is more likely to lead to injury than stiffness. We can, however, consider how much tension we are holding in our tissues by using joint mobility techniques. If we rotate our foot, for example, we can get a sense of how much tightness is held in the tissues of the lower leg. Marjariasana (Cat/Cow) highlights the tightness in the tissues of our back. Notice that I do not say '*muscles*'. Tension is held in the fascia or connective tissue, which includes the wrapping of muscles. You can find a rounded sequence on joint mobility in the vāta sequence in Appendix 2. Ultimately, it is better to consider the body as a whole in every movement, because nothing works in isolation, so it is best to include all movements in a daily practice.

COOLING

When you are running yoga classes in the middle of summer or live in a hot climate, it makes total sense to have 'cooling' as a theme. Cooling includes all pitta-pacifying practice (see Appendix 3).

These are the key practices:

- Sitāli
- Seetkari
- Chandra bheda
- Gentle, mindful movement that focuses on stretching, squeezing and toning the abdominal area like gentle back bends, forward bends and twists
- Cultivating a devotional mindset
- Cultivating gratitude
- Cultivating a sense of surrender and letting go.

REVITALIZING FOR LONGEVITY (RASĀYANA)

Revitalizing therapy or Rasāyana Chikitsā is a big part of the Āyurvedic protocol. Āyurveda uses panchakarma to cleanse the body, followed by a period of careful dieting and herbs to rebuild the body. We can adapt this idea to our yoga practice by considering the approach taken in the *HYP*. The 'bindu' is an area at the back of the head, which was believed to be the seat of amrita, or nectar. It was believed that as our lives progress, the amrita gradually trickles down our digestive tract and gets burned up by jaṭhara agni (digestive fire). This was thought to be a measure of how long we would live and was the whole basis of tantric claims of greater longevity through the practice of inversions.

The term used in the *HYP* is Viparīta Karaṇī. In modern practice, we consider this to be similar to Sarvāṅgāsana (Shoulder Stand) because this is how it was interpreted by the Iyengar and Bihar schools of yoga. However, there is no mention of this in the *HYP*. Viparīta Karaṇī means 'Inverted pose'. This means that it can actually be any pose that puts the body in an inverted state, including semi-inversions like Adho Mukha Svanāsana (Downward Facing Dog pose) and standing forward bends. Obviously, this is not the same experience because the marma points in the head and neck are not stimulated, but for the purposes of this discussion, it is possible to build a class around it. Teaching full inversions would obviously not be suitable for beginners but may be an interesting enquiry for more experienced students.

Certain marma points can also be included in this theme (see Chapter 8).

NOURISHING

The idea of a nourishing practice draws upon the Āyurvedic concept of brmhana, which literally means 'bulk increasing'. We usually hold that quality of lightness or laṅghana over brmhana because a light body is more likely to be disease-free, but a closer study of Āyurveda will reveal that in the case of illness and burnout, the body and soul need to be nourished and rebuilt back to health. Both yoga and Āyurveda actually subscribe to the idea of 'preserving' energy rather than spending it, because if we waste all our energy, we end up being too tired to pursue the highest goal of Mokṣa or spiritual liberation.

Many of us are much more tired than we think. In the absence of tea and coffee, you may realize that you have been running on empty and need to nurture yourself.

This kind of class should involve long passive holds in āsanas that require little physical effort, such as:

- Eka Pada Rājakapotāsana (King Pigeon pose)
- Supta Pādāṅguṣṭhāsana (Reclining Hand to Big Toe pose)
- Salamba Bhujaṅgāsana (Sphinx pose/Supported Cobra pose)

- Jānu Śīrṣāsana (Head to Knee pose)
- Vīrāsana (Hero's pose), also known as Vajrayana (Thunderbolt pose)
- Paścimottānāsana (Seated Forward Bend)
- Mālāsana (Garland pose)
- Viparīta Karaṇī (Inverted pose: supported with legs up the wall)
- Sarvanana (Shoulder Stand: supported on a chair)
- Uttānāsana (Standing Forward Bend).

There are many other poses you can use that will passively open up the body in different ways, but these are the ones I usually work with.

LAṄGHANA (LIGHTENING)

This is the opposite principle to nourishing or brmhana. To cultivate the experience of lightness, it is useful to work with upward-moving poses and clearing exercises.

Here are some suggestions of standing poses.

- Vīrabhadrāsana 1 (Warrior 1)
- Vīrabhadrāsana 3 (Warrior 3)
- Tiryaka Tāḍāsana (Swaying Palm Tree pose)
- Vṛkṣāsana (Tree pose)
- Naṭarājāsana (Dancer's pose)
- Trikoṇāsana (Triangle pose)
- Ardhā Chandrāsana (Half Moon pose: triangle balance)
- Adho Mukha Vṛkṣāsana (Down Facing Tree or Handstand)

If you have ropes in your yoga studio, you can use them to create more lightness in Adho Mukha Svanāsana (Downward Facing Dog pose), as well as forward bends and other inversions.

ROOTING THROUGH THE FEET (VĀTA PACIFYING)

I teach this theme a lot because I find that students are not well connected to the ground. Our feet are stuck in shoes all day long. We walk on concrete and then when we get home, we wear slippers and walk on carpet. At no point do we allow our feet to truly make contact with the ground. I find it useful to try and make contact with a natural surface every day; perhaps a stony or sandy beach, grass or the earth itself. I appreciate there are many barriers to this. You may be living in a city and have little access to nature, or even if you do, the climate may be too cold. At least you can free your feet for the duration of a yoga class. I started using a cork mat and noticed that the health of my feet improved immediately. Practising on rubber mats is very practical but not that pleasant. Rooting through the feet can be a great way to pacify vāta doṣa and get people out of their heads. It is a variation on the theme of grounding.

Obviously, a yoga class on rooting will include a lot of standing poses, but the more we experiment with the idea of leading with the feet, the more we realize that engaging the feet can in fact facilitate all posture work. We learn to engage the body from the ground upwards.

Here are some key postures for working with rooting.

- Tāḍāsana (Mountain pose)
- Vīrabhadrāsana 1 (Warrior 1)
- Vīrabhadrāsana 3 (Warrior 3)
- Vṛkṣāsana (Tree pose)
- Trikoṇāsana (Triangle pose)
- Ardhā Chandrāsana (Half Moon pose: triangle balance)
- Parsvottanasana (Intense Side Stretch)
- Prasārita Pādottānāsana (Wide Legged Forward Bend)
- Uttānāsana (Standing Forward Bend)

DṚṢṬIS (FOCUSED GAZING)

This concept has always been around but it was popularized by the Aṣṭāṅga vinyasa style of practice. It is an application of Patanjali's practice of Dhāraṇā (concentration). Using focal points during your āsana practice is a good way of steadying the mind, so it is very useful for the management of vāta doṣas. A Dṛṣṭi can be external or internal. It is best to consider internal work separately, because keeping the eyes open or closed has a different impact.

Here are the key Dṛṣṭis.

- A point on your body:
  - Tips of the fingers and toes
  - Tip of the nose
  - Eyebrow centre
  - Navel.
- A point nearby:
  - A point on the wall or floor
  - An object
  - A drawn symbol
  - A candle flame.

ASTROLOGICAL SYMBOLISM (PRAKṚTI)

This is a slightly odd theme that very few teachers work with. As a trained astrologer, I have occasionally indulged in astrological correspondences because I have found that it helps people understand something about their Prakṛti or innate constitution. There are many ways of working with astrology.

- **Get students to imagine the characteristic behaviour of an animal as described by astrology:** Of course, we are not trying to understand the animal itself. It would be like trying to understand a human being by learning about fairy-tale caricatures. We are using our imagined version to understand something about the characteristics of a sun in a certain sign.

- **Work with astrological elements:** Earth, water, fire, air. The expressions of the four elements are very similar to those described in Āyurveda, so we are building on the same idea.
- **Pair work and group work:** What happens when you group all fire signs together or all Capricorns together? This helps you and your students identify and celebrate a certain kind of modus operandi.

TABLE 10.7: WORKING WITH ASTROLOGY

Astrological sign	Ruling element and quality	Symbolism
Aries (22 March–21 April)	Cardinal fire	Ram
Taurus (22 April –21 May)	Fixed earth	Bull
Gemini (22 May–21 June)	Mutable air	Twins
Cancer (22 June–21 July)	Cardinal water	Crab
Leo (22 July–21 August)	Fixed fire	Lion
Virgo (22 August–21 September)	Mutable earth	Virgin maiden
Libra (22 September–21 October)	Cardinal air	Scales
Scorpio (22 October–21 November)	Fixed water	Scorpion
Sagittarius (22 November–21 December)	Mutable fire	Centaur
Capricorn 22 (December–21 January)	Cardinal earth	Goat
Aquarius (22 January–21 February)	Fixed air	Waterbearer
Pisces (22 February–21 March)	Mutable water	Fish

SENSES

This is a very useful tantric technique that helps us attune our awareness to our internal as well as external senses. You may recall that right relationship with the senses is one of the Āyurvedic definitions of health. There is huge scope for working with the senses. Here are just some ideas.

- **Sound:** Tibetan bowls, rāga music, mantra (see Chapter 12), Antar Mouna (inner silence), Nada yoga (sound yoga).

- **Vision:** Chitākāśa (mind space), colours, Dṛṣṭis, symbols, chākras, crystals.
- **Touch:** Marma points, crystals, pair work, wall, floor, different textures.
- **Smell:** Essential oils, incense, imagined smells.
- **Taste:** Imagined tastes, chocolate or raisin meditation, current taste in the mouth, deciding on the main rasa or taste of a food, Khechari mudrā.

MEDITATION ON THE PRĀṆIC BODY

There are many ways of working with the prāṇic body. We have touched on several techniques already, but here is a summary of key approaches.

- Chākra trigger points (Kṣetra) that run up the midline of the front torso
- Chākra points in the spine
- Marma points
- Imagination of colour, symbol, quality, etc.
- Yogic meridians
- Mudrā
- Bandha
- Ujjayi breath with visualization.

Chapter 11

YOGA NIDRĀ WITH ĀYURVEDIC THEMES

The practice of Yoga Nidrā as we know it today was formulated by Swami Satyananda Saraswati in the 1970s.[1] It is based on older tantric practices but was adapted into a system that takes you through a carefully developed therapeutic process.

Yoga Nidrā is performed in a supine position and is loosely translated as psychic sleep. This is because one appears to be asleep during the practice, but the consciousness has withdrawn to a much deeper level.

Yoga Nidrā employs some very simple but powerful techniques. Unlike many practices, there is no concentration involved. You are only required to listen and feel, to connect to the words of the speaker and notice what feelings arise. You may not even pick up every word the speaker says. It gets harder and harder to do so, the deeper you go into relaxation. However, it is important that one maintains awareness of the speaker's voice and what arises from within. One should resist the temptation to intellectualize the process – let it 'wash over you' so to speak. This state of allowing is an important part of the therapeutic process.

Many people fall asleep during a session. Strictly speaking, this should be resisted because, once you lose connection with the speaker, the process cannot be as beneficial.

From my experience, students who can't help falling asleep are usually

---

1 Satyananda Saraswati, Swami (1976). *Yoga Nidrā*. (Fifth edition.) Bihar: Bihar School of Yoga.

very tired from their lives, so I do not insist on wakefulness. However, it is useful to at least set an intention to do stay awake.

Yoga Nidrā can easily be adapted to integrate Āyurvedic themes. It is a fixed format but the theme for every practice will vary, like any other yoga class. Many subtle practices can be integrated into a Yoga Nidrā, including chākras, mantra, breathing and visualization. If you want to keep the practice congruent with an Āyurvedic theme, you can select appropriate symbols, sensations and states and build them in.

There are seven stages to Satyananda's system.

1. Preparation.
2. Resolve or Saṅkalpa.
3. Rotation of consciousness.
4. Awareness of breath.
5. Feelings and sensations.
6. Visualization.
7. Repetition of Saṅkalpa.

Stage 1: Preparation

This is an essential stage for a successful Yoga Nidrā. There are two phases of preparation.

1. Comfort and receptivity

Making sure:

- You will not be disturbed.
- You are comfortable enough to remain physically still.
- You have enough support for your neck, back and knees.
- Your head is in the direction of the speaker.
- Your body is in contact with the floor and nothing else.
- You can hear the instructions clearly.

Once you are physically prepared, the final part of this phase is to prepare yourself mentally.

Mentally repeat: 'I am about to practise Yoga Nidrā. I will remain awake and aware.'

2. Relaxing the body

One of the main aims of Yoga Nidrā is to relax the body so much that the mind is able to enter a hypnogogic state, where it wavers between sleep and wakefulness. This is known as the alpha state, where the mind becomes very relaxed and receptive.

If we let ourselves fall asleep, our mind moves into what is called a delta state, where we are no longer conscious, so it is harder to work with our subconscious drives. On the other end of the scale, in everyday life, the mind is usually in a beta and sometimes gamma state, so it is not possible to work with the deeper layers of our mind.

It is only when our brain emits alpha or theta waves that change is possible, because we are still conscious. This is why it is important to stay awake and aware. Remaining in this state is one of the most difficult skills to cultivate but, with persistence, it is possible.

Here are some key techniques for relaxing the body.

- Contact between the body and the floor.
- Movement of the breath through the nostrils.
- Spatial awareness.
- Awareness of distal and local noises (Antar Mouna).
- Counting the breaths down to zero. (This can also be done in the breathing section but it is a good technique for relaxation.)
- Observing the contents of the mind space (Chitākāśa).

Stage 2: Resolve, or Saṅkalpa

Saṅkalpa means 'resolve' or 'resolution'.[2] It is a key component in achieving your goals. When you have managed to relax the mind and body sufficiently, it is time to plant an idea. Originally, the future tense was used when articulating a resolve, but current research suggests that it is better to prompt the mind into imagining that something has already been achieved rather than holding it in the future. Instead of saying, 'I will fulfil my spiritual potential,' it is better to say, 'I am fulfilling my spiritual potential.' This is important because setting a resolution in the future keeps it in the future. You want to condition your mind to experience a desired state in the present. Even if it is only imagined, it is important to actually feel what it would be like to fulfil your goal. This is a very powerful tool for attracting what you want.

It is also best to avoid goals that are too outwardly oriented. Happiness is a feeling that arises from within and though that feeling is somewhat dependent on the external conditions, Yoga Nidrā works in reverse. Once you embody the feeling of happiness and immerse your mind in the imagined fulfilment of a goal, external circumstances will eventually change to match your inner state. It seems counterintuitive but it works because it is drawing upon the powerful law of attraction.

The power of imagination

Try to get to the heart of what you are really seeking.

- If you want to be famous, for example, you are really seeking love and validation, so that is the feeling you should try and cultivate during the practice.

- If you want to be rich, you are really seeking a state of unconditional abundance. What would that feel like? Focus on that.

- If you are looking for a relationship, you are really seeking unconditional love and intimacy. What would that feel like if you already had it?

---

2 *Ibid.* (p.22)

> Try to get to the heart of what you are really seeking.

There is no shame in desiring. Kāma, or desire, is one of the pillars of Āyurveda and is the most natural thing in the world. Without desire, we are not motivated to live, but what we think we want does not always match up with what we need. All we need to do is focus on the feeling we are looking for and leave the rest to god. Our God-Self or Ātman sits on a higher perch, so sometimes we just need to trust that everything is as it should be.

Stage 3: Rotation of consciousness

This is based on areas of heightened sensitivity around the body. Satyananda refers to the homunculus man, a representation of what a person would look like if their body were built according to areas of higher and lower sensitivity. Many of these areas are also marma points, so we will build that aspect into the work too. There are longer and shorter versions of this, depending on how much time you have. The longer versions are really good training for the mind, but I have used a shorter version here that is more suitable for a general yoga class, where a Yoga Nidrā session is unlikely to be more than 20 minutes.

Here is the standard order of instruction.

> Right thumb, second finger, third finger, fourth finger, little finger, palm of the hand, back of the hand, wrist, lower arm, elbow, upper arm, shoulder, armpit, waist, hip, right thigh, knee, calf, ankle, heel, sole of the foot, top of the foot, right big toe, second toe, third toe, fourth toe and little toe.
>
> Left thumb, etc. …
>
> Right shoulder, left shoulder, right shoulder blade, left shoulder blade, right buttock, left buttock, the spine, the whole of the back together.
>
> Top of the head, forehead, right eyebrow, left eyebrow, the eyebrow centre, right eyelid, left eyelid, right eye, left eye, right ear, left ear, right cheek, left cheek, nose, tip of the nose, right nostril, left nostril, upper lip, lower lip, chin, jaw, throat, right collarbone,

left collarbone, right side of the chest, left side of the chest, centre of the chest, navel, abdomen, lower abdomen.

Whole of the right leg, whole of the left leg, both legs together, whole of the right arm, whole of the left arm, both arms together, whole of the back, whole of the front, whole of the head, whole of the body.

Stage 4: Awareness of breath

The breath is our main vehicle for bringing prāṇa into the body. Vāta controls the mind, and prāṇa is the essence of vāta. Therefore, we need to spend some time with the breath during Yoga Nidrā. Most of the time we are breathing spontaneously and noticing how it becomes less and less perceptible the more we relax. However, we can also practise psychic variations of prāṇāyāma whilst lying down and this can have a powerful effect on the mind.

- **Breathing between the navel and the throat:** The front channel (arohan) is used in several tantric practices. We imagine breathing up and down the front of the body along an imagined silver thread that connects the navel to the throat. This technique works with the chākras and the prāṇic body. The navel is the main Kṣetra or field of influence for Manipūra Chākra (actually at the L3/4 vertebral level, which aligns with the navel) and the throat is the Kṣetra for Vishuddhi Chākra. This method seeks to better integrate our prāṇic field.
- **Psychic breathing:** This is one of my favourite Yoga Nidrā practices. You imagine you are practising alternate nostril breathing. Some students are flummoxed by this and try to use their fingers, but you will be amazed how effective it is. By simply imagining you are breathing in through one nostril and out through the other, it eventually feels like it is happening. The mind comes into balance because the solar and lunar poles of the prāṇic body come into balance (ida: lunar; piṅgala: solar). A balanced mind is able to relax yet remain clear at the same time.

Stage 5: Feelings and sensations

This stage may need a little care. We want our students to go deep and to feel that they have agency and control over what they allow themselves to think and feel, but we don't want to evoke anything that is too difficult to handle. We invite students to imagine sensations from memory: sensations of heat-cold/heavy-light/pain-pleasure and so on.

The purpose of this is to impress on them the idea that the mind has a part to play in what we experience. When we are in physical pain caused by an accident or trauma, it is unhelpful to say that it is all in the mind, and we need to care for ourselves. However, if we are caught in a cycle of chronic long-term pain, it is useful to know that we can use our mind to bring some relief. We must never get habituated to pain, because it eventually finds its way into our identity and we can no longer remember who we were before the pain started. This exercise is empowering because it demonstrates that the mind has the power to alter perception of mental and physical states.

Here is an example of the kind of instruction you might give.

> Recollect a time when your body was very cold, so cold that it was shivering.
>
> Recollect a time when your body was hot, boiling hot, so hot that you were sweating.
>
> Recollect a time when your body was in pain, agonizing pain. [Keep this short.]
>
> Now recollect a time when your body was immersed in bliss, every cell, smiling with pleasure.
>
> Your body feels heavy, so heavy that you are sinking into the ground.
>
> Your body feels light. As light as a feather. So light that you are floating off the ground.

Āyurveda

This is a good section to help your students cultivate a guna or quality in their bodies.

- To pacify vāta, focus on the qualities of heaviness, sweetness, warmth, tenderness, kindness, joy and softness
- To pacify pitta, focus on coolness, calm, sweetness, surrender and acceptance
- To pacify kapha, focus on lightness, heat, motivation, drive, spaciousness and detachment.

Marma points

This is a good section to build Marma Chikitsā (marma therapy) into the practice. This is useful and relevant because marmani are junctions between the physical body and the prāṇic body, so they can be used as a gateway between the two sheaths. Yoga Nidrā is about healing the whole person and works on all aspects of the prāṇic and mental sheaths.

If you are unfamiliar with marma points, this may not be something you wish to include. Read Chapter 8 to gain an understanding of how to identify and use marma points in general yoga practice before attempting to include them in Yoga Nidrā. The key thing is to make sure that students of all levels can feel where the marma points are. There is no point in referring to obscure locations. Refer to very obvious points like the head, heart, lower abdomen, feet and hands. All major joints are marma zones, including the knees, elbows, shoulders and spine. The face and head are full of marma points too. Using marmani to enhance the healing process is a fascinating field and will definitely enrich your teaching once you have gained a proper understanding of it.

Stage 6: Visualization

This section can be very enjoyable to experience if you can stay awake that long! Satyananda liked to use archetypal images that evoked heightened spiritual feelings, including temples, crosses, images of sages, nature and so on. Using archetypal images is important because symbol is a powerful way of bypassing the conscious mind. Fairy tales are built on archetypes, for example, which is why they have universal appeal. It is best to use images that have a universal appeal and will be readily accessible to most cultures. A word of warning: not all of your students will have the same associations as you. Symbols are deeply personal, but if you provide a rich enough landscape, you should be able to appeal to everybody. I have used a variety of symbols over the years, including:

- Astrological signs and symbols (animals, shapes, etc.) (see Chapter 10)
- Chākra correspondences (colours, shapes, animals) (see Appendix 6)
- Nature and natural events like sunset, sunrise, full and crescent moons, blue sea, golden sun, red earth, green grass, lush forest, animals, mountains and so on.

Āyurvedic symbolism

Here is another opportunity to bring Āyurveda into the practice. You can be very specific about the types of symbols you choose to use. Here are some examples of how to use symbols to pacify the doṣas.

- **Vāta:** Warm earth, soft green grass under your feet, a soothing sunset, a warm embrace, soft golden light, the love of a furry cat, a mother's love.
- **Pitta:** The cool ocean, a full moon in a clear, star-filled sky, a green emerald, a blue sapphire, a snow-capped mountain.
- **Kapha:** A lion, a cheetah, a warm sunrise, golden sand, a flying eagle, endless space.

All these symbols are designed to evoke a relationship that can help to pacify a particular doṣa. Take a look at the 20 gunas (see Chapter 7) and see if you can think of your own. You can evoke sensations through images, but the sensation must come from an archetypal symbol: mother, cat, water, sun, moon, etc. If it is a part of nature, it is allowed. If it comes from a very old tradition, it too is allowed. Crosses, squares, circles, pentagrams, etc. are all sacred geometry.

Stage 7: Repetition of Saṅkalpa

It is important to repeat the Saṅkalpa three more times just before the practice finishes, to reinforce the resolve. That way, the idea is impressed in the manas (lower mind) as well as the deeper mind (buddhi).

- A Saṅkalpa for someone with vāta imbalances should focus on overcoming fear and feeling nurtured and safe.
- A Saṅkalpa for someone with pitta imbalances should focus on kindness, compassion and acceptance.
- A Saṅkalpa for someone with kapha imbalances should focus on love, positivity and drive.

Choosing to teach Yoga Nidrā

Yoga Nidrā takes a lot of practice and training. Many yoga teachers take elements of it and think that they are teaching it when, in fact, they are just teaching a guided relaxation. They are not the same. Yoga Nidrā is a tantric tool designed to heal and transform. It is powerful. Work with an experienced teacher for a while before you decide to teach it yourself. The best teachers of Yoga Nidrā are from the Bihar School of Yoga. Don't learn from someone who does not have a track record of proper training and understanding. You will be cheating yourself and your students of a more authentic experience.

> Yoga Nidrā is a tantric tool designed to heal and transform. It is powerful.

Yoga Nidrā scripts

Stages 1, 3 and Finish are always the same and I have boxed them for easy reference.

Yoga Nidrā sample script for pacifying vāta

STAGE 1: PREPARATION

Get ready for Yoga Nidrā. Make sure you will not be disturbed. Please switch off your mobile phone now. Lie on your back with your head facing the speaker, your legs apart and your arms away from your body, palms facing upwards. Make sure you will be warm and comfortable throughout the practice and take any props you need to support your back, knees and neck. Make any final adjustments you need to make now so that you can lie as still as possible for the next 20 minutes. Close your eyes and keep them closed for the duration of the practice.

Now, mentally repeat: 'I am about to practise Yoga Nidrā. I will remain awake and aware. I am about to practise Yoga Nidrā. I will remain awake and aware.'

Become aware of the contact points between your body and the ground. Really tune in to these contact points and feel your body sinking into the ground. There is no limit to how much you can give yourself to the ground. Feel your body getting heavier and heavier through these contact points. Your body is still. Your body is stable. You are completely relaxed. Your feet are relaxed. Your hands are relaxed. Your body is relaxed. Your eyes are sinking into their sockets. Your tongue is settling onto the floor of your mouth. Your forehead is soft, your throat is soft, your jaw is loose. You are completely relaxed. Your legs feel heavy. Your arms feel heavy. Your body feels heavy. Your head feels heavy. You are letting go. It is time to let yourself go, to allow yourself to be held and nurtured.

Become aware of the breath flowing in and out of your nostrils. The natural breath flowing in and out, in and out, in and out. Every time you breathe out, you feel yourself getting more relaxed.

Now, start to count your breaths down from ten to zero. Inhaling and exhaling on ten, inhaling and exhaling on nine, all the way down to zero. If you lose count, start again; it doesn't matter.

Pause... The next breath will be the last breath you count.

STAGE 2: SAṄKALPA

It is time to make your Saṅkalpa. Imagine a version of yourself that is full of joy and enthusiasm. Free from fear and optimistic. Mentally repeat:

> I am free to express and to share the life and energy that I have with the world.
>
> I am free to express and to share the life and energy that I have with the world.
>
> I am free to express and to share the life and energy that I have with the world.

STAGE 3: ROTATION OF CONSCIOUSNESS

Now, it is time for the rotation of consciousness. I will be moving quite fast through all parts of your body. Try to touch each part I name with your mind, but you must keep your body absolutely still.

Your right-hand thumb, second finger, third finger, fourth finger, little finger, palm of the right hand, back of the hand, wrist, lower arm, elbow, upper arm, shoulder, armpit, right side of the waist, right hip, right thigh, right knee, right calf, right ankle, heel, sole of the foot, top of the foot, right big toe, second toe, third toe, fourth toe and little toe.

Your left thumb, second finger, third finger, fourth finger, little finger, palm of the left hand, back of the hand, wrist, lower arm, elbow, upper arm, shoulder, armpit, left side of the waist, left hip, left thigh, left knee, left calf, left ankle, heel, sole of the foot, top of the foot, left big toe, second toe, third toe, fourth toe and little toe.

Right shoulder, left shoulder, right shoulder blade, left shoulder blade, right buttock, left buttock, the spine, the whole of the back together.

Top of the head, forehead, right eyebrow, left eyebrow, the eyebrow centre, right eyelid, left eyelid, right eye, left eye, right ear, left ear, right cheek, left cheek, nose, tip of the nose, right nostril, left nostril, upper lip, lower lip, chin, jaw, throat, right collarbone, left collarbone, right side of the chest, left side of the chest, centre of the chest, navel, abdomen, lower abdomen.

Whole of the right leg, whole of the left leg, both legs together, whole of the right arm, whole of the left arm, both arms together, whole of the back, whole of the front, whole of the head, whole of the right side of the body, whole of the left side of the body, the whole of the body, the whole of the body.

STAGE 4: AWARENESS OF BREATH

Bring your awareness back to your breath and pay attention to the quality of your breath.

Pause

Make your breath as smooth as you can.

Pause

Now, even out the breath so the inhalation is the same length as the exhalation.

Pause

Now, imagine you are breathing in through the left nostril on a count of four and breathing out through the right nostril on a count of four.

Then breathe in through the right on four and breathe out through the left on four.

Inhale left, two, three, four.

Exhale right, two, three, four.

Inhale right, two, three, four.

Exhale left two, three, four.

Continue at your own pace for a few rounds.

Pause

Now, imagine you are breathing up and down the spine.

Up and down the spine.

Up and down.

Up and down.

Pause

STAGE 5: FEELINGS AND SENSATIONS

Now, bring your awareness to your body and imagine that it is made of solid rock. Solid and stable. Strong and unyielding.

Now, imagine your body is filled with warm liquid undulating inside you. You are soft and pliable, like a bag of water.

Now, imagine that your heart is a golden egg circulating golden light all around your body. Filling every corner of your body with its golden rays. You are so full of light that your cells are radiating. You are a luminous body of light.

STAGE 6: VISUALIZATION

Now, visualize the following.

- A tall mountain overlooking a vast blue sea
- Warm red earth under your feet
- Lying on soft green grass
- A golden sunset
- A warm sunrise
- An affectionate white cat
- A loving mother
- A warm breeze
- A golden beach
- The sound of waves
- Red clouds
- A burning candle
- Stars at night
- A full moon
- Swimming in warm water

- A dolphin
- A meadow
- Cows roaming in a field
- A sweet peach.

STAGE 7: REPETITION OF SAṄKALPA

Now it is time to repeat your Saṅkalpa. Mentally repeat the following three more times:

> I am free to express and to share the life and energy that I have with the world.
>
> I am free to express and to share the life and energy that I have with the world.
>
> I am free to express and to share the life and energy that I have with the world.

FINISH

Now, start to become aware of yourself lying on the floor.
Become aware of yourself breathing.
Start to wriggle your fingers and toes.
Rotate your ankles and wrists.
Gently move your head from side to side.
Bend your legs into your chest and roll over to the right side.
Stay on the right side for a few breaths.
Now slowly sit up, keeping your eyes closed.
Make Anjali mudrā (prayer position) with your hands in front of your chest and repeat the mantra Om once.
Yoga Nidrā is now complete.
Hari Om Tat Sat.

Yoga Nidrā sample script for the chākras

STAGE 1: PREPARATION

See box on page 216.

STAGE 2: SAṄKALPA

It is time to make your Saṅkalpa. Tune in to your heart space and imagine you are looking into your soul. What is your heart's true desire? What feeling are you looking to experience? Hold on to that feeling and know that it is already available to you right now. Is there a word that encapsulates that feeling? Perhaps a colour? If there is, repeat that word three times, imagining the colour at the same time. If there are no words or colours, then stay with the feeling.

STAGE 3: ROTATION OF CONSCIOUSNESS

Now it is time for the rotation of consciousness. See box on pages 217–18.

STAGE 4: AWARENESS OF BREATH

Bring your awareness back to your breath and pay attention to the quality of your breath. Can you cultivate a very gentle, barely perceptible ujjayi breath that only you can hear, like listening to the sound of a seashell?

Pause

Imagine you are breathing up and down the spine, a gentle breeze blowing up and down the spine.

Now, imagine you are breathing in and out of the pelvic floor, visualizing a deep red.

Now, you are breathing between the pubic bone and the sacrum, visualizing an orangey-red colour.

Now, you are breathing between the navel and the spine, visualizing a fiery yellow colour.

Now, you are breathing between the chest and the spine, visualizing a bright green colour.

Now, you are expanding the bluey breath in the throat, so it is felt throughout the neck.

Now, you are breathing in and out of the point between your eyebrows, visualizing the colour of indigo.

Feel the breath passing through the eyebrow centre and out of the back of the head on the inhalation and then back the opposite way on the out breath.

Finally, visualize a rainbow as you breathe in and out of the top of your head.

Long pause

STAGE 5: FEELINGS AND SENSATIONS

Now, bring your awareness back to Mūlādhāra Chākra in the pelvic floor and see if you can recollect a time when you felt financially insecure. Now, cultivate the sensation of complete trust and faith. You are well looked after, and all will be well.

Pause

Now, bring your awareness back to Svādishthāna Chākra in the sacral area and recollect a time when you were obsessively attached to something or someone.

Pause

Now, cultivate the sensation of detachment and freedom. You are already complete. You can let go of desire at any time and enjoy every moment for what it is. You already have everything you need.

Pause

Now, bring your attention back to Manipūra Chākra in the navel and the spine and recollect a time when you felt completely powerless and weak.

Now, cultivate the sensation of strength and infinite power. You have all the power you need to make your way through life without hurting anyone else. You believe in yourself completely.

Pause

Now, bring your awareness back to Anāhata Chākra in the heart space and the spine and recollect a time when you felt hurt or let down by love.

Now, cultivate that loving feeling again and know that it is everywhere all the time and is not conditional. You have all the love you need.

Pause

Now, bring your attention back to the throat and the neck and recollect a time when you didn't feel heard or felt that you'd lost your voice or your ideas were ignored.

Now, imagine yourself speaking with such love and truth and everyone stopping to listen to you, and trust that you will always be heard by those who need to connect with you.

Pause

Now, bring your attention to Ājñā Chākra at your eyebrow centre and the centre of your head and recollect a time when your life was full of darkness and ignorance.

Now, cultivate the satisfaction of wisdom, forgive yourself for your mistakes and thank life for showing you the way.

STAGE 6: VISUALIZATION

Now, visualize the following.

- A white elephant.
- A white elephant standing on a yellow cube.
- A white elephant standing on a yellow cube with a flower painted on its side. The flower has four bright red petals.
- A friendly crocodile swimming in a quiet lake. It is night-time. There is a crescent moon lying on its back. Along the edge of the lake are orange flowers with six petals.
- A fierce-looking ram in a dusty yellow field. The field is triangular in shape. Growing in the fields are marigolds with ten yellow petals.
- A sensitive deer in a magical forest full of trees with star-shaped leaves. The leaves have six points and glow. On the ground are growing plants with 12 leaves spreading out to catch the sun's rays.

- An elegant swan gliding over a still, circular, deep-blue lake. Along the edges are flowers with 16 petals. Four on top, four on the bottom, four on the right and four on the left.
- An eagle soaring through the air. Its wings are a striking indigo colour.

STAGE 7: REPETITION OF SAṄKALPA

It is time to repeat your Saṅkalpa. Tune back in to your heart space and imagine you are looking into your soul. What is your heart's true desire? What feeling did you identify as your greatest need? Hold on to that feeling again and know that it is already available to you right now. Repeat any word that arose from that feeling and hold any colour in your mind for three breaths. If there were no words or colours, stay with the feeling for three more breaths.

FINISH

See box on pages 220–21.

—Chapter 12—

TEACHING MANTRA FROM AN ĀYURVEDIC PERSPECTIVE

Mantra is a word, sound or combination of sounds that are repeated to aid concentration or meditation. There is a lot of myth and folklore around mantra and it is arguably one of the oldest forms of yoga. Mantras are made up of Sanskrit sounds. They can be in the form of a single syllable, known as a Bīja mantra, or a combination of sounds in the form of a phrase.

Mantra phrases usually pay homage to Hindu deities, but their use goes way beyond our current understanding. Sanskrit is considered to be a divine language in the sense that when uttered, it is believed to raise our overall vibration and uplift us. Hindu pundits devote their lives to learning verses from the *Vedas* and use them in community rituals. Many traditional Āyurvedic clinics, including the one I've used in Hyderabad, have a resident pundit who blesses the Āyurvedic process every day. It is part and parcel of authentic Āyurvedic treatment.

It is thought that a true mantra is one that has been used to achieve the ultimate enlightened state. You may be given a mantra by an enlightened master, or one of his initiates, as a segue into spiritual life. It is, however, also possible to work with different mantras for mundane purposes.

Mantra and Āyurveda

Āyurveda recommends using mantra to work on the mind. It considers mantra to be a powerful tool for overcoming mental imbalances and making the mind stronger. It is one of the few purely yogic practices recommended by Charaka. Frawley *et al.*[1] say that mantra means 'that which saves [trayati] the mind [manas]'.

Mantra in yoga classes

Mantra work is usually quite cursory in general yoga classes. Chanting Om at the start and end of a yoga class is part of the Sivananda and other monastic traditions, but you rarely get mantra in western yoga classes inspired by householder traditions like Krishnamacharya or Iyengar.

From an Āyurvedic perspective, mantra work is important because it is considered to be a major tool in managing the mind. Sivananda always used to say that mantra was an effective way of purifying the mind, but I'm not sure what this really means or whether it is relevant in modern life. I do subscribe to the idea that it changes your perspective and patterns of thinking if you practise regularly. It raises positivity and brings about greater clarity. In this sense, it raises sattva guna. The mind becomes a higher-functioning tool and there is less chance of making errors of judgement or Prajñāparādha.

There are so many ways of using mantra. As most students of yoga can only experience techniques through general classes, I think it is important to adapt techniques so that students can at least try them out. If they want to go on to learn more, they can attend workshops. When you translate mantras into English, they sound a bit silly, so I don't recommend this. If you have a problem with chanting in Sanskrit, it might be better to use English affirmations instead.

Mantras can be used in yoga classes to:

- Pacify doṣas
- Increase ojas

1 Frawley, D. (1998). *Āyurveda and the Mind*. Delhi: Motilal Banarsidass. (p.225)

- Improve mental functioning
- Cultivate greater insight
- Help clear mental blockages
- Induce bliss and wellness
- Increase vitality and fortitude.

It is beyond the scope of this book to explore mantra in detail, but I will comment on the most commonly taught mantra, Om, the Bīja mantras associated with the chākras and how to use mantra with Sūrya Namaskara (Sun Salutation).

The mantra Om

Om is made up of four parts. A-U-M-0. The last part, '0', represents silence. In Sanskrit grammar, *A* and *U* are combined to make up the sound *O* but they can equally be chanted separately.

Om is the most sacred of all mantras because it represents the All, the entirety of the cosmos. Some teachers say it is the original sound of the universe that emerged with the Big Bang. Om should not be used as a personal mantra on its own because the energy it holds is too vast, but it has traditionally been used to start and end classes. It is usually part of a longer mantra that pays homage to one of the Hindu deities, for example, Om namah Shivaya (paying homage to Shiva).

Other popular mantras

- Om namo narayanaya (Vishnu)
- Om dum durgaye namaha (Durga)
- Om aim saraswatiye namaha (Saraswati)
- Om sri maha Lakṣmīye namaha (Lakṣmī)
- Om gam ganapatiye namaha (Ganesha)

Mantras of the chākras[2]

Many yoga teachers who have been trained in mantra will occasionally work with the main Bīja mantras associated with the chākras. When working with mantra, it is useful to bring in other senses so the mind is consumed with the various facets of the vibration.

TABLE 12.1: BĪJA MANTRAS OF THE CHĀKRAS

Bīja mantra	Element	Colour	Shapes
Laṃ	Earth	Deep red	Yellow square
Vaṃ	Water	Orange	White crescent moon
Raṃ	Fire	Yellow	Red upward-pointing triangle
Yaṃ	Air	Green	Smoky six-pointed star
Haṃ	Space	Blue	Dark blue circle
Om	Mind	White or indigo	A small point

Mantra in Sūrya Namaskara (Sun Salutation)

Sun Salutation, or Sūrya Namaskara, is one of the most common practices taught in yoga classes. It was popularized in the early 20th century and has been adopted by several yoga schools. It is a sequence of connecting āsanas that start and end with Tāḍāsana (Mountain pose) and is often used to warm up the body in classes. It is possible, however, to use Sūrya Namaskar as a complete practice in itself.

Using mantra and applying an ujjayi breath during the practice of Sūrya Namaskara (Sun Salutation) can have a profound effect. The sequence can take on a sacredness that is otherwise lost. There are many different forms of Sūrya Namaskara. In the Sivananda traditions, 12 common names of the sun are mentally repeated during the course of a long ujjayi in breath or out breath as each āsana is performed. Combining the ujjayi breath (prāṇāyāma) with the mental repetition of mantra and the 12 āsanas makes this a complete Haṭha yoga practice in itself. Namaha is everywhere in mantra and means 'salutations to'.

2 Sivananda, Swami (1991). *Kundalini Yoga*. (Ninth edition.) Tehri-Garhwal: Divine Life Society.

Here are the 12 movements with their corresponding mantras; each āsana is performed with the repetition of a mantra during the inhalation or exhalation.

TABLE 12.2: MANTRA IN SŪRYA NAMASKARA[3]

	Posture	Instruction	Mantra and breath	Concentration
1	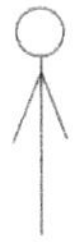 Tāḍāsana (Mountain pose)	Hands in Anjali mudrā (prayer position). Eyes closed. Even breathing. Wait for an exhalation to begin.	Exhale Om mitraya namaha	Anāhata Heart centre Mitraya means 'one who is friendly to all'
2	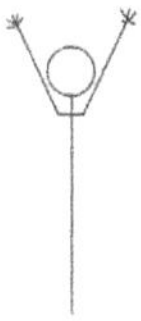 Hasta Uttānāsana (Raised Arm pose)	Inhale: raise the arms above the head and gently arch the whole back (not just the lumbar).	Inhale Om ravaye namaha	Vishuddhi Throat chākra Ravaye means 'the shining one'
3	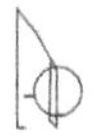 Uttānāsana (Standing Forward Bend)	Exhale: come into a forward bend with slightly bent legs.	Exhale Om sūryaya namaha	Svādishthāna Sacral chākra Sūrya is the dispeller of darkness
4	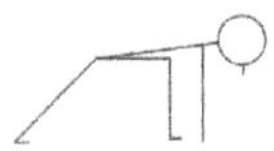 Anjaneyasana (Low Lunge) Lunge backwards	Inhale: lunge the left/right leg back and lift the chest without throwing the head back.	Inhale Om bhanave namaha	Ājñā Eyebrow centre Bhanave is the one who illuminates
5	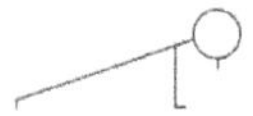 Phalakasana (Plank pose)	Hold the breath in Phalakasana.	Hold breath Om khagaya namaha	Manipūra Navel chākra Khagaya is the one who moves through the sky

3 Adapted from Satyananda Saraswati Swami (1973). *Sūrya Namaskar*. Bihar: Bihar School of Yoga.

6	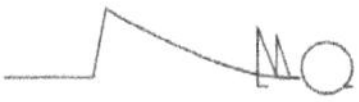 Astanga Namaskara (Eight-Point pose)	Exhale: lower the knees, chest and forehead to the ground.	Exhale Om pushne namaha	Manipūra Navel chākra Pushne is the giver of nourishment and fulfilment
7	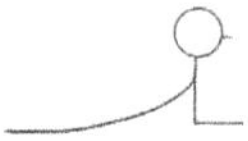 Bhujaṅgāsana (Cobra pose)	Inhale: gentle Bhujaṅgāsana (Cobra pose), leading with the chest. This can be replaced with Urdhva Mukha Śvānāsana (Upward Facing Dog) if preferred.	Om hiran-yagarbhaya namaha	Svādishthāna Sacral chākra Hiranyagarbha means 'the golden egg': the cosmic womb of creation
8	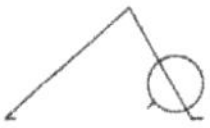 Adho Mukha Svanāsana (Downward Facing Dog pose)	Exhale: press the hands down and draw the buttocks back into Adho Mukha Svanāsa-na (Downward Facing Dog pose).	Om marichaye namaha	Vishuddhi Throat chākra Maricha is the son of Brahma who brings the golden rays of the sun
9	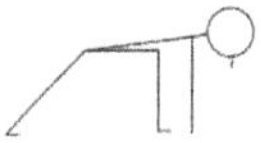 Anjaneyasana (Low Lunge) Lunge forwards	Inhale: lunge the right/left foot forward between the hands.	Om adityaya namaha	Ājñā Eyebrow centre Aditi is the cosmic mother
10	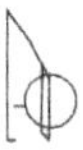 Uttānāsana (Standing Forward Bend)	Exhale: both feet together in a standing forward bend.	Om savitre namaha	Svādishthāna Sacral chākra Savitre is the stimulating power of the sun
11	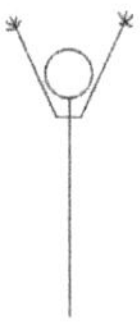 Hasta Uttānāsana (Raised Arm pose)	Inhale: raise the arms above the head and gently arch the whole back.	Om arkaya namaha	Vishuddhi Throat chākra Arkaya means 'the one who is worthy of praise and glory'
12	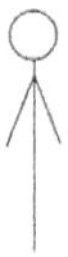 Tāḍāsana (Mountain pose)	Exhale: hands in Anjali mudrā (prayer position) in Tāḍāsana (Mountain pose).	Om bhaskaraya namaha	Anāhata Heart chākra Bhaskara is the giver of wisdom and cosmic illumination

Chapter 13

THE ĀYURVEDIC JOURNEY

We have reached the end of this leg of the journey. You now have some idea of the cosmic dream that imagined our existence and then hid itself away from us so that we could discover its magnificence all for ourselves.

The Āyurvedic journey is rich with adventure and it was never meant to be travelled without its trusted partner: yoga. The two together make a formidable team because, with their combined skills, they are able to maintain a healthy body and mind and a contented soul. The greatest of all crimes are committed out of ignorance (avidya), our inability to not only understand the true nature of reality but also to feel it in our hearts.

When we awaken to our heart's intelligence, we realize that we do not live in isolation. We live in communities and depend on each other every day. It is sometimes easy to get lost in the lofty ideas of yoga and Āyurveda and forget that the real truth of things stands right before us. The proverbial seekers of treasure spend their whole lives seeking out the mysteries of life and eventually, often too late, realize that it was both within them and all around them all along. We sometimes shun the abundance of love offered to us unconditionally in favour of greater challenge, risk and danger, but realize that the true courage that makes a person is that of surrendering a frightened yet tenacious ego to a truth that is greater than the sum of separate ego-driven parts.

We are carried through a story in the compassionate arms of the great mother, who keeps reminding us to eat properly, get enough sleep, do exercise and manage our stress so that we can live our lives with greater passion and energy. There is work to be done, but there is really only one job: to overcome ignorance and live in harmony with each other and with nature. Everything else is an untruth and ultimately harms us.

Take these teachings to your students, your family, your friends. Embody their principles in your own life and keep yourself steadfast in the face of mockery and scorn. With yoga and Āyurveda on your side, you are in the winning team, and over time you and everyone who knows you will realize it.

Hari Om Tat Sat

Tarik

GLOSSARY OF SANSKRIT TERMS

Sanskrit term (saṃskṛta)	Meaning
Adhipati	Lord
Adho	Below
Adho Mukha Svanāsana	Downward Facing Dog pose
Ādinātha	First Lord
Agadatantra	Toxicology
Agni	Fire
Agra	Tip
Ājñā	Understanding
Ākāśa	Space
Ālocaka	Eyes
Āma	Uncooked
Anāhata Chākra	Unstruck; heart chākra
Ānandamayakośa	Bliss sheath
Aṅgulī	Width of middle finger
Annamayakośa	Food sheath
Antar Mouna	Inner silence
Anuloma	In the natural direction
Apāna	Downward flow of vāta
Ardhā	Half
Ardhā Chandrāsana	Half Moon pose

Sanskrit term (saṃskṛta)	Meaning
Artha	Treasure
Āsana	Posture
Aṣṭāṅga	Eight limbed
Aṣṭāṅga Saṅgraha	One of the three major works of Āyurveda
Atharvā	Name of fourth Veda
Atipravṛtti	Excessive flow
Atiyoga	Excess
Ātman	Soul/God-Self
Avalaṃbaka kapha	Kapha in the chest
Ayoga	Unsuitable
Āyurveda	Knowledge of life
Baddhakoṇāsana	Cobbler's pose
Balā	Strength
Bandha	Lock
Basti	Bladder/lower abdomen
Bhastrikā	Bellows breath
Bheda	Breaking, separation
Bhrājakapitta	Pitta in the skin (related to lustre)
Bhujaṅgāsana	Cobra pose
Bhūtavidyā	Demonology
Bīja	Seed
Bodhaka kapha	Kapha located in the mouth (taste perception)
Brāhmamuhūrta	Two muhurtas, equivalent to 1 hour and 36 minutes before dawn
Bṛhat	Solid, lofty
Bṛṃhaṇa	Building
Buddhi	Intellect or wisdom mind
Cala	Moving
Caraka Saṃhitā	The definitive classic written around 2nd century BCE
Chākra	Wheel, vortex
Chikitsā	Treatment
Chitta	Mind stuff, perception

Darśana	Seeing, philosophy
Dhairyam	Calm, composed
Dhāraṇā	Steadiness
Dharma	Right action
Dhātu	Tissue; bodily support
Dinacaryā	Daily routine
Dīpana	Kindling
Dīrgha	Long lasting
Doṣa	Functional entity of the body prone to vitiation
Drava	Juice, fluid
Dṛṣṭi	Glance, focused gaze
Duḥkha	Aversion
Eka Pada Rājakapotāsana	King Pigeon pose
Gaṇḍūṣa	Gargle
Garbhadhana	Supports the womb
Graha	Demon, grab, seize
Gulpha	Ankle
Guna	Quality, attribute
Guru	Heavy; sage
Haṃ	Bīja mantra for ākāśa
Harṣā	Joy
Haṭha	Force
Hṛdaya	Heart
Indrabasti	Marma point on calf and wrist
Indriya	Sense organ
Jālandhara	One of the 84 Siddhas; refers to the throat lock in the *HYP*
Jānu	Knee
Jaṭhara	Abdomen, belly
Jiva	Life
Jivana	Vitalizing
Jyoti	Light
Kāma	Desire
Kapālabhātī	Shining skull practice from the *HYP*

Sanskrit term (saṃskṛta)	Meaning
Kapha	One of the three doṣas
Kapila	Main teacher of Sāṃkhya philosophy
Kara	The cause of
Karmendriya	Organ of action
Kaṭhina	Hard
Kaṭi	Hips (also refers to sacral marma)
Kaumārabhṛtya	Paediatrics
Kāya	Human body
Kāyacikitsā	General medicine
Khara	Rough
Kledaka kapha	Kapha in the stomach
Kṛkāṭikā	Back of the neck (refers to a marma point)
Kṣetra	Body; territory; field; refers to the field of influence in tantric meditation
Kṣipra	Rapid; quick acting; refers to a marma point between the thumb and index finger
Kumbhaka	Retention
Kūrca	Bundle; refers to marma points at the ball of the foot
Kūrcaśiras	Marma point at the root of the thumb and head of the heel
Kūrpara	Elbow
Laghu	Light
Lakṣmī	Hindu goddess of abundance and good fortune
Laṃ	Seed mantra for the root chākra
Laṅghana	Lightening; reducing
Lepa	Covering; anointing
Lohitākṣa	Marma point in the armpit
Mahānārāyaṇa	The Great Narayana; a common medicated oil used for pain in Āyurveda
Mālāsana	Garland pose
Manda	Dull
Mandāgni	Sluggish digestion
Māṇibandha	Marma point on the wrist band
Manipūra Chākra	City of jewels; navel chākra

Manomayakośa	Mind sheath
Mantra	Incantation or phrase used for meditation
Marma	Vital part
Marmani	Vital parts
Mātrosna	Optimal body temperature
Matsyendrāsana	One of the 84 classical poses: Seated Spinal Twist
Medhākara	Promotes intelligence
Mithyā	Incorrect
Mokṣa	Spiritual liberation
Mṛdu	Soft
Mudrā	Gesture
Mukha	Mouth
Mūlādhāra Chākra	Root chākra
Nābhi	Navel
Nādi	Channel
Nāsā	Nose
Nāsikāgra	Nose tip
Nasya	Nasal (errhine) therapy
Naṭarājāsana	Dancer's pose (Naṭarāja posture)
Nāvāsana	Boat pose
Nidrā	Sleep
Ojas	Vital fluid
Pāchakapitta	Pitta in the digestive tract
Pāchana	Cook
Pakti	Digested; ripened
Paścimottānāsana	Seated Forward Bend
Piṅgala	Subtle channel that carries solar energy
Pitta	One of the three doṣas
Poṣaṇa	Nourishing
Prabhā	Lustre
Pradīpikā	Light
Prajñāparādha	Crime against wisdom
Prakṛti	The latent and manifest universe; unique constitution

Sanskrit term (saṃskṛta)	Meaning
Prāṇa	Animating principle
Prāṇa	Vital force; one of the five sub-doṣas of vāta
Prāṇamayakośa	Prāṇic sheath
Prāṇāyāma	Expansion and control of prāṇa
Prasāda	Essence
Prasārita Pādottānāsana	Wide Legged Forward Bend
Prema	Love
Prīṇana	Pleasing; gratifying
Pūraṇa	Filling up; used to fill a cavity
Rāga	Colouring; classical Indian music
Rajas	One of the three yogic gunas; kinetic energy of the universe
Rakta Mokṣana	Blood letting
Raṃ	Seed mantra for navel chākra
Rañjaka pitta	Pitta in the blood
Rasa	Taste; lymph; blood plasma
Rasāyana	Rejuvenation
Rig Veda	Oldest of the four *Vedas*
Ṛtucharyā	Seasonal routine
Rūkṣa	Dry
Sacchidānanda	Existence, consciousness and bliss
Sādhakapitta	Pitta located in the brain
Sahasrāra Chākra	Thousand-petalled chākra
Śālākya	Surgery
Śālākyatantra	Supraclavicular diseases
Śalyatantra	Surgery
Śam	A seed mantra representing wellness and health
Samāgni	Balanced digestive fire
Samāna	One of the five sub-doṣas of vāta
Śamana Chikitsā	Pacifying treatment
Sāṃkhya	One of the six Indian philosophies
Sanātana	Eternal
Sandhyā	Junction; joint

Sāndra	Thick
Saṅgraha	Compilation
Saṅkalpa	Resolution
Śaṅkha	Conch shell; marma point at the temples
Sarvāṅgāsana	Shoulder Stand
Sattva	One of the three yogic gunas, representing balance and harmony
Śaurya	Prowess; heroism
Śirovasti	Pouring oil on the head (Āyurvedic treatment)
Śīrṣāsana	Headstand
Śīta	Cold
Sitāli	Cooling breath
Slakshna	Smooth
Śleṣaka kapha	Kapha located in the joints
Snehana	Oleation
Snigdha	Oily
Śodhana	Purification
Śrīṃ	Seed mantra for the goddess Lakshmi, representing abundance and wellness
Śṛṅgāṭaka	Where four roads meet; marma point at back of the throat
Srotas	Channels
Sthāna	Residence; sacred place
Sthāpanī	Marma point at the eyebrow centre
Sthira	Stable
Sthūla	Gross
Sukha	Pleasure; comfort; happiness
Sūkṣma	Minute; subtle
Supta Pādāṅguṣṭhāsana	Reclining Hand to Big Toe pose
Sūrya	Sun
Suśruta Saṃhitā	Compilation written by the surgeon Suśruta
Sūtrasthāna	First book in all three works of Āyurveda that deals with basic principles
Svādishthāna Chākra	Dweller of the self; sacral chākra

Sanskrit term (saṃskṛta)	Meaning
Swatmarama	Author of the *HYP*
Taittirīyopaniṣad	*Upaniṣad* that mentions the five sheaths
Talahṛdaya	Marma point at centre of the sole of the foot and palm of the hand
Tamas	One of the three gunas; darkness; ignorance
Tapas	Heat; austerity
Tarpaka kapha	Kapha located in the head
Tejas	Essence of pitta doṣa
Tīkṣṇa	Sharp
Tīkṣṇāgni	Overactive agni caused by excess pitta
Tiryaka Tāḍāsana	Swaying Palm Tree pose
Trikoṇāsana	Triangle pose
Udāna	One of the five sub-doṣas of vāta
Ujjayi	Victorious breath
Upadhātu	Subsidiary tissue
Upaniṣad	Sacred Indian texts spanning thousands of years
Uṣṇa	Hot
Utkaṭāsana	Powerful pose
Uttānāsana	Standing Forward Bend
Utthita Pārśvakoṇāsana	Extended Side Angle pose
Vājīkaraṇa	Virility treatment
Vaṃ	Seed mantra for the sacral chākra
Vaṃana	Emesis
Varṇa	Colour; complexion
Vāta	One of the three doṣas
Vijñānamayakośa	Wisdom or intuitive sheath
Vikṛti	Imbalance
Villoma	Against the grain; backwards
Vimārga gamanam	Moving in the wrong direction; bad road
Viparīta Karaṇī	Inverted pose
Vīrabhadrāsana	Warrior pose
Vīrāsana	Hero's pose

Virechana	Purgation therapy
Vīrya	Potency
Viṣa	Poison
Viśada	Clear; non slimy; shiny
Viṣamāgni	Irregular digestion
Vishuddhi Chākra	Throat chākra; purification
Vṛkṣāsana	Tree pose
Vrukka	Kidney
Vyāna	One of the five sub-doṣas of vāta; controls general circulation
Yaṃ	The bīja mantra of the Anāhata Chākra (heart)
Yantra	Geometric symbol used for meditation

—*Appendix 1*—

ĀYURVEDIC CONSTITUTIONAL ASSESSMENT (PRAKṚTI)

Tick or circle the characteristics that best describe you as you have been for most of your life. If two characteristics in different boxes apply equally, tick **both**. Only give **one tick per box**, regardless of how many words there are in the box. If you have been very changeable, tick vāta. **Leave out** any you don't know the answer to or that don't apply to you. There are several characteristics in a single box; they may not all apply to you, but some will. Be as honest as you can. There is no better or worse. When counting up, make sure you give **two points** for every ticked box in the **physical characteristics** section and **one point per ticked box** for the rest. Count **downwards** (not across) and write the grand totals at the end.

TABLE A1.1: ĀYURVEDIC CONSTITUTIONAL ASSESSMENT

		Vāta	Pitta	Kapha
Physical characteristics (give two points per ticked box as you count each column downwards)				
1	**Height**	Unusually short or tall.	Medium (for your race).	Tall and sturdy or short and stocky.
2	**Weight**	Light. Difficulty putting on weight.	Moderate. No problem gaining or losing weight.	Heavy. Find it hard to lose weight.
3	**Frame**	Light. Thin. Narrow hips and shoulders.	Medium.	Large. Broad shoulders. Big hips.

4	**Joints**	Prominent. Knobbly. Cracking.	Normal. Well proportioned.	Big. Deep set. Well lubricated.
5	**Musculature**	Slight. Difficulty putting on muscle.	Medium. Well proportioned.	Solid. Lots of muscle mass.
6	**Skin**	Thin. Dry. Darkish. Cold. Rough. Cracked. Wrinkles. Prominent veins.	Fair. Soft. Lustrous. Warm. Many moles and freckles. Prone to acne.	Thick. Oily. Pale or white. Cold. Smooth. Moist.
7	**Hair**	Thin. Dark. Coarse.	Fine. Soft. Fair. Red-dish. Early greying or balding.	Plentiful. Thick. Very wavy. Lustrous. Oily.
8	**Shape of face**	Long. Angular.	Heart shaped. Sharp contours.	Large and round. Fat. Soft contours.
9	**Neck**	Thin. Very long or very short.	Average. In proportion.	Solid. Tree-trunk like.
10	**Nose**	Crooked. Small. Narrow.	Neat. Pointed. Average.	Large. Rounded. Oily.
11	**Eyes**	Small. Narrow. Sunken. Dark. Dull. Small eyelashes.	Average size. Light. Easily inflamed. Piercing. Intense. Fine eyelashes.	Large. Prominent. Liquid. Thick eyelashes. Attractive. Prone to crust easily.
12	**Teeth**	Irregular. Protruding. Receding gums.	Medium sized. Yellowish.	White. Big. Strong gums.
13	**Mouth**	Small.	Medium.	Large.
14	**Lips**	Thin. Narrow. Tight. Dry.	Average. Soft. Red.	Big. Full. Firm. Lush.
15	**Legs**	Thin. Excessively long or short. Prominent knees. Small hard calves.	Medium. Well shaped and proportioned. Loose calves.	Large. Stocky. Meaty calves.
16	**Voice**	Breathy. Hoarse. Chatty.	Concise. Impatient	Slow. Cautious. Reserved.
17	**Feet**	Small. Thin. Dry. Rough. Bony.	Medium. Soft. Pink.	Large. Fleshy.
Psychological states (give one point per ticked box)				
18	**Thinking**	Superficial with many ideas. More thoughts than deeds.	Precise. Logical. Good planner. Dominant. Sharp.	Calm. Slow. Cannot be rushed. Good organizer.
19	**Memory**	Good short term. Poor long term.	Very good. Quick to recall.	Good long term but takes time to learn.

		Vāta	Pitta	Kapha
20	**Deep beliefs**	Frequently changing according to mood. Indecisive.	Very strong convictions. Passionate. Opinionated.	Steady beliefs that don't change easily. Stubborn.
21	**Emotional tendencies**	Fearful. Anxious. Insecure.	Angry. Judgemental.	Greedy. Possessive.
22	**Work preference**	Creative. Varied and social.	Intellectual. Cerebral. Goal oriented.	Caring. Physical. Practical.
23	**Lifestyle**	Erratic. Irregular. Always on the go.	Ambitious. Driven.	Steady and regular. Can get stuck in a rut.
24	**Speech**	Quick. Talkative.	Sharp. Argumentative.	Slow. Quiet.
25	**Dreams**	Vivid or easily forgotten. Flying.	Passionate. Usually remembered. In colour.	Cool. Calm. Uneventful
26	**Vulnerable sense organ**	Hearing (sensitive to loud noises).	Sight (sensitive to bright light).	Touch and smell (sensitive to the touch and smell of others).
Metabolic tendencies (give one point per ticked box)				
27	**Menstruation**	Irregular cycles. Scanty dark blood.	Regular cycles. Bleed for a long time. Bright red blood.	Regular periods. Average light-coloured blood.
28	**Urine (abnormal)**	Scanty. Colourless. (Darkish when unwell).	Profuse. (Burning when unwell.)	Moderate. (Mucus/whitish when unwell.)
29	**Bowel movements**	Variable. Sometimes dry and hard, sometimes loose. Gas.	Abundant. Loose. Yellowish. Burning sensation.	Moderate. Well formed. Mucus.
30	**Sweat**	Scanty. No smell.	Copious. Hot. Strong fleshy smell.	Moderate and consistent. Cold. Pleasant smell.
31	**Appetite**	Variable. Erratic.	Strong. Sharp.	Low. Regular.
32	**Thirst**	Forgets to drink.	Excessive thirst.	Little thirst.
Physiological functions (give one point per ticked box)				
33	**Activity**	Quick. Fast. Unsteady. Erratic. Hyperactive.	Motivated. Purposeful. Goal oriented.	Slow. Steady. Unruffled.

34	**Strength**	Quick to start but poor endurance.	Medium. Strong mental determination.	Good endurance once warmed up.
35	**Sex drive**	Quick to get aroused. Prone to overindulgence. Low endurance.	Hot-blooded. Goal focused. Get angry if not gratified.	Steady desire. Slow to get aroused. Good endurance.
36	**Sleep**	Light. Variable. Easily disturbed. Prone to insomnia 2am–6am.	Consistent. Prone to insomnia and hunger 12am–2am.	Heavy and deep.
37	**Climate preference**	Warmth at all times. Lose strength in the winter.	Prefer cooler climates. Easily irritated by heat and strong light.	Prefer dry warm climates but generally not bothered.
38	**Disease tendency**	Weak immunity. Nervous system. Pain. Arthritis. Mental disorders.	Medium resistance. Spreading diseases. Infections. Fevers. Inflammation.	Good resistance. Prone to congestive disorders. Respiratory system. Swelling.
39	**Circulation**	Poor. Variable.	Good. Warm.	Medium. Prone to swelling.
40	**Pulse**	Fast. Slippery. Like a snake.	Medium. Jumpy. Like a frog.	Slow. Smooth Like a swan.
Grand totals				

Appendix 2

SEQUENCE FOR MANAGING VĀTA DOṢA

Vāta is like the wind. Unpredictable, restless, light and cooling. When vāta is out of balance, we should try to introduce the opposite qualities into our practice. Eventually, although perhaps not at first, our practice should be gentle, still, mindful and nurturing. The breath should be even, smooth and deep to help calm the body and mind. Postures are held steadily for a short time (six breaths) and should not be tiring. It is better to repeat a challenging posture than hold it for a long time. The practice should end with a generous relaxation and some deep abdominal breathing.

TABLE A2.1: SEQUENCE FOR MANAGING VĀTA DOṢA

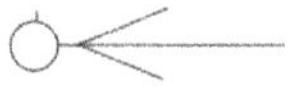	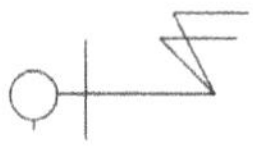	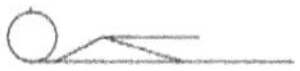	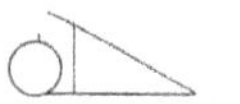	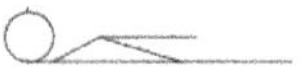
Savasana (Corpse pose). Abdominal breathing.	Jaṭhara Parivritti (Revolved Abdomen pose). Full breathing into the ribcage	Apānasana (Wind Relieving pose). Bending the knees into the body on an out breath	Supta Pādāṅguṣṭhāsana (Reclining Hand to Big Toe pose). Gently lengthening the backs of the legs. A belt can be used.	Sucirandhrasana (Eye of Needle pose). Opens the front hip.

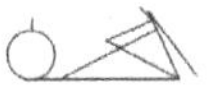		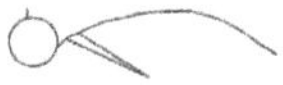	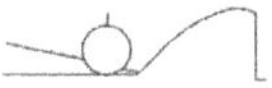	
Sucirandhrasana (Eye of Needle pose) other leg.	Catch the feet and pull down both legs into an upside-down squat.	Setu Bandhasana (Bridge pose). Engages the legs and extends the spine. Lift on exhalation.	Open chest variation.	Apānasana (Wind Relieving pose) counterpose.
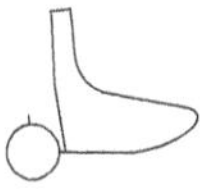	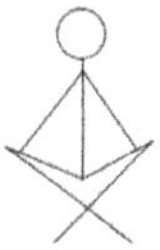		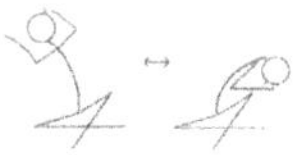	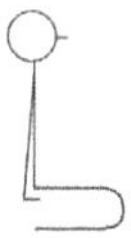
Rolling back and forth over the spine. Loosens the vertebrae.	Sukhāsana (Easy pose). Steady breathing.	Baddhakoṇasana (modified) (Half Cobbler pose).	Side stretching and twisting on exhalation.	Kneeling and lifting the knees to stretch the tops of the feet.
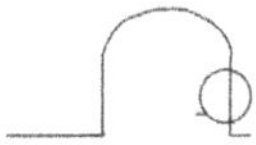	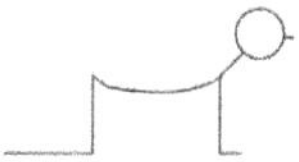	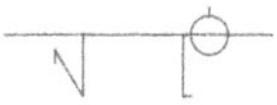	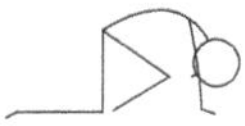	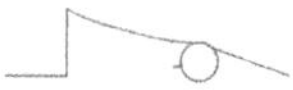
Marjariasana (Cat). Inhale.	Marjariasana (Cow). Exhale.	Vyaghrasana (Tiger pose). Extend on exhalation.	Inhale.	Shashankasana (Hare pose). Rest.
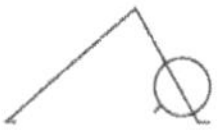		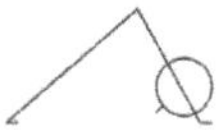		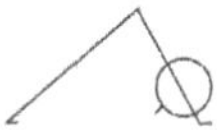
Adho Mukha Svanāsana (Downward Facing Dog pose). Keep legs bent if necessary.	Lunges. Stay for six breaths.	Adho Mukha Svanasana (Downward Facing Dog pose). Keep legs bent if necessary.	Salamba Bhujaṅgāsana (Sphinx pose/ Supported Cobra pose). Hold for six.	Adho Mukha Svanasana (Downward Facing Dog pose). Keep legs bent if necessary.

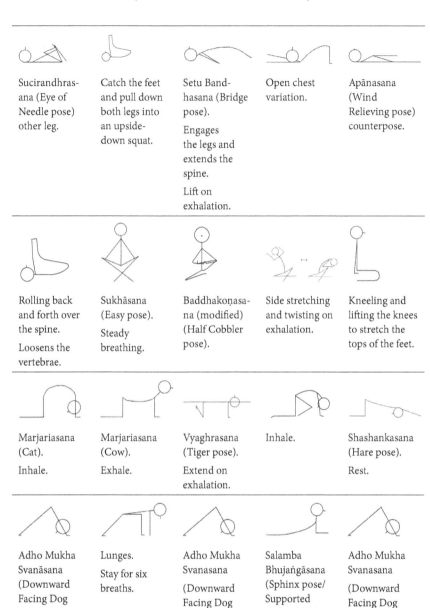

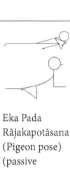

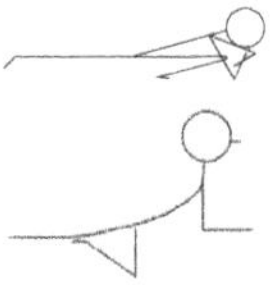	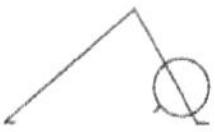	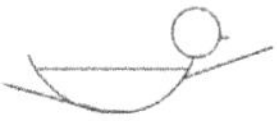	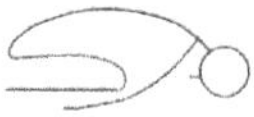	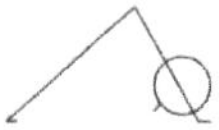
Eka Pada Rājakapotāsana (Pigeon pose) (passive and active variations).	Dog counterpose.	Single-leg Shalabhasana (Locust pose). Be careful with back pain.	Balāsana (Child's pose). Counterpose.	Adho Mukha Svanāsana (Downward Facing Dog pose) to lead into standing poses.
	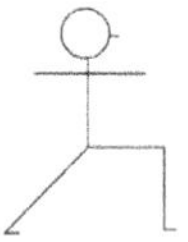	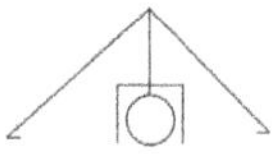	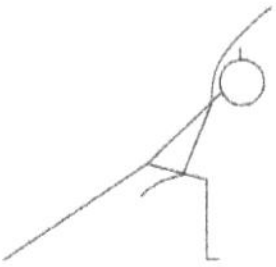	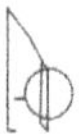
Tāḍāsana (Mountain pose). Be still for six breaths. Side stretches (three on each side).	Vīrabhadrāsana 2 (Warrior 2).	Prasārita Pādottānāsana (Wide Legged Forward Bend).	Utthita Pārśvakoṇāsana (Extended Side Angle pose).	Uttānāsana (Standing Forward Bend).
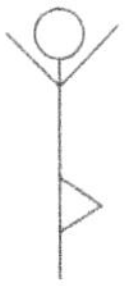	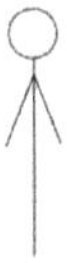	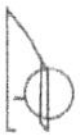	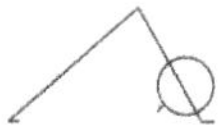	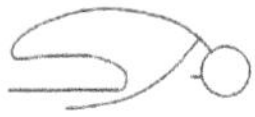
Vṛkṣāsana (Tree pose).	Tāḍāsana (Mountain pose).	Forward bend.	Adho Mukha Svanāsana (Downward Facing Dog pose).	Balāsana (Child's pose).
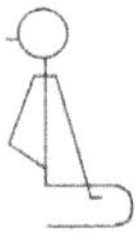	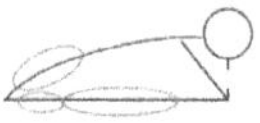	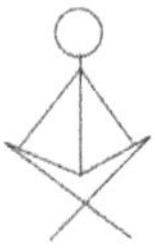	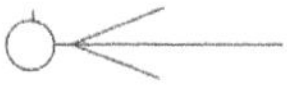	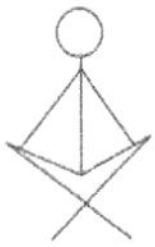
Seated twist.	Jānu Śīrṣāsana (Head to Knee pose). Seated forward bend.	Baddhakoṇāsana (Cobbler's pose).	Savasana (Corpse pose). Deep abdominal breathing.	Quiet sitting.

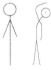

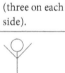

Options

- You can repeat a posture more than once if you have the energy.
- You can add more standing postures, such as Trikoṇāsana (Triangle pose) and Parsvottanasana (Intense Side Stretch).
- You can repeat the Sūrya Namaskara (Sun Salutation) several times – up to six on each side.
- You can add a short Dhanurasana (Bow pose) after Shalabhasana (Locust pose).
- You can mix up the sequence. You may prefer to do the standing poses first and then all the seated and supine work towards the end.
- You can lie with the legs up the wall instead of conventional Savasana (Corpse pose).

Your own notes:

—Appendix 3—

GENTLE PITTA-BALANCING SEQUENCE

Pitta doṣa is driven by fire, and water is its container. Fire needs fuel to burn and when properly managed it can produce tremendous creative flair, energy and radiance. It depends on earth and water qualities to keep it under control because it cannot do this for itself. We cultivate coolness, calm and a sense of surrender to help the fire dissipate so the body and mind can settle. Focus on sustaining a deep diaphragmatic breath, even during twists and rotations, to maximize the squeezing and toning of the abdominal area.

Sit quietly for a few breaths and cultivate a smooth, soothing, sibilant breath using the mantras śam and śrīṃ. With even exhalation, use śam and śrīṃ to keep the body and mind cool during the practice.

TABLE A3.1: GENTLE PITTA-BALANCING SEQUENCE

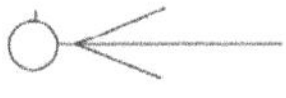	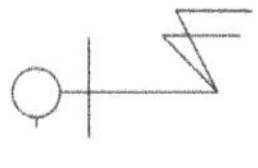	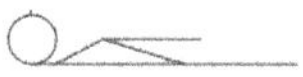	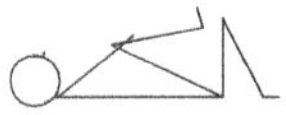	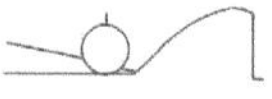
Savasana (Corpse pose).	Jaṭhara Parivritti (Revolved Abdomen pose).	Apānasana (Wind Relieving pose).	Apānasana (Wind Relieving pose) – single leg.	Setu Bandhasana (Bridge pose).

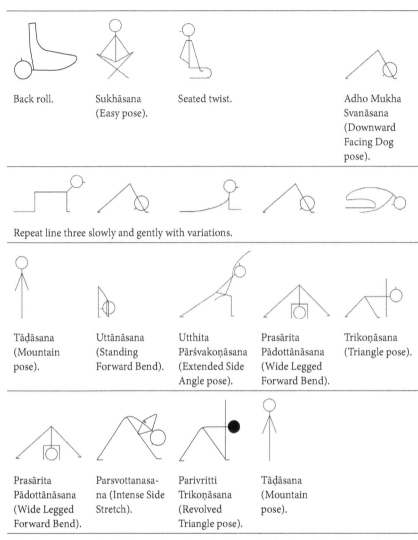

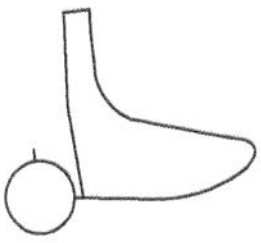
Back roll.

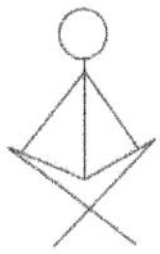
Sukhāsana (Easy pose).

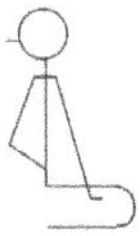
Seated twist.

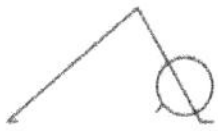
Adho Mukha Svanāsana (Downward Facing Dog pose).

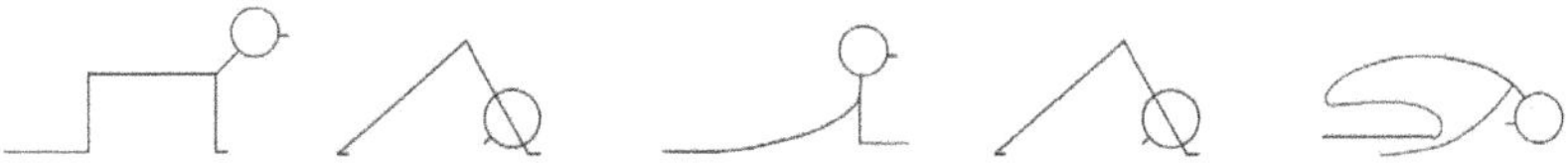

Repeat line three slowly and gently with variations.

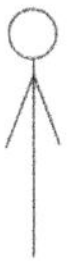
Tāḍāsana (Mountain pose).

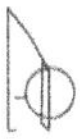
Uttānāsana (Standing Forward Bend).

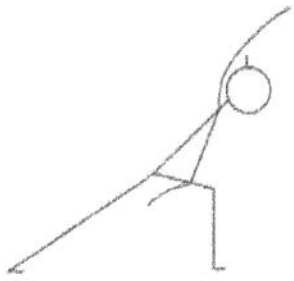
Utthita Pārśvakoṇāsana (Extended Side Angle pose).

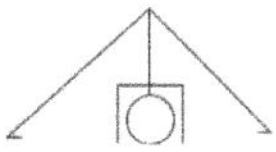
Prasārita Pādottānāsana (Wide Legged Forward Bend).

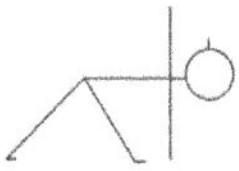
Trikoṇāsana (Triangle pose).

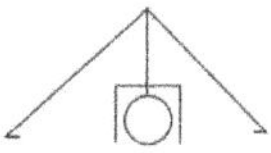
Prasārita Pādottānāsana (Wide Legged Forward Bend).

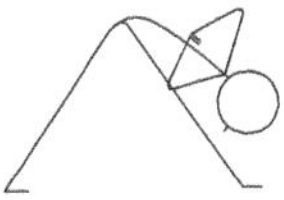
Parsvottanasana (Intense Side Stretch).

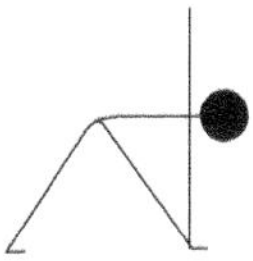
Parivritti Trikoṇāsana (Revolved Triangle pose).

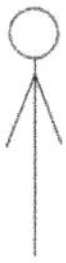
Tāḍāsana (Mountain pose).

Standing postures should focus on length and rotation with short steady holds up to half capacity.

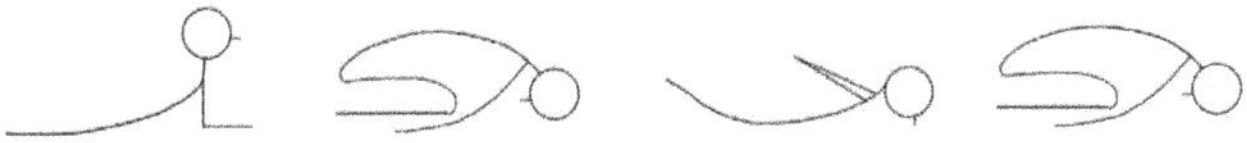

Back bends should focus on gentle spinal extension and abdominal stretch and tension release.

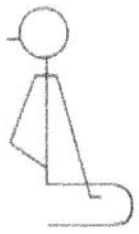 Matsyendrāsana (Seated Spinal Twist).	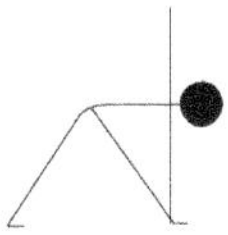 Ardhā Matsyendrāsana (Half Spinal Twist).	Twists should focus on the squeezing and toning of the abdominal area with a full diaphragmatic breath.
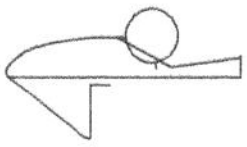	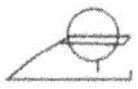	Seated forward bends. Kindle agni but reduce pitta. Use the śam breath on the exhalation.
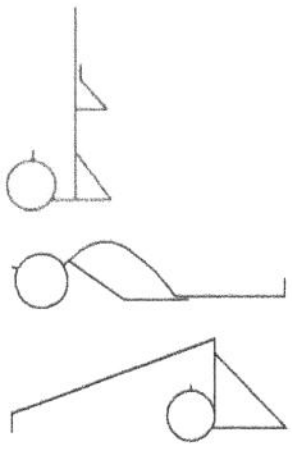		Sarvāṅgāsana (Shoulder Stand) sequence to finish and a medium length Savasana (Corpse pose).

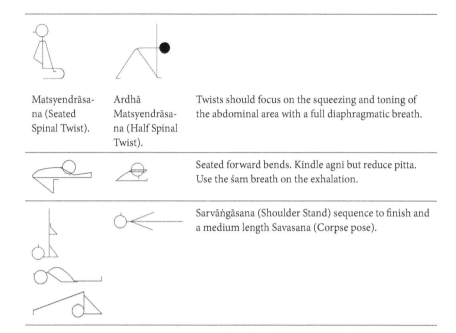

—Appendix 4—

SEQUENCE FOR BALANCING KAPHA DOṢA

Principles of practice for kapha doṣas

Energetics: Kapha has a tendency to heaviness, solidity, cold and torpidity. When using āsana to balance kapha, we are ultimately looking to creating more lightness, warmth and dynamism in the body. It is difficult to create this from the outset, so it is important to start gently and gradually build momentum and warmth in the body. Then, it is possible to work very strongly over a longer period of time.

We are looking to promote the qualities of buoyancy, lightness, warmth, spaciousness in the joints, chest and lungs, and good postural integrity to promote a fullness of breath.

Kinaesthetic focus: The upper band around kapha's primary seat is the primary focus initially. This means that there will be greater emphasis on the stomach, chest and upper back, extending into the head, sinuses, lungs and throat. The sub-doṣas of kapha include the saliva in the mouth (bodhaka), lubrication in the joints (śleṣaka), the heart and lungs (avalaṃbhaka), the brain (tarpaka) and, of course, the stomach (kledaka). Any practice that brings attention to these areas may be considered beneficial to the balance of kapha, including marma points and mudrā practices like Khechari mudrā.

TABLE A4.1: SEQUENCE FOR BALANCING KAPHA DOṢAS

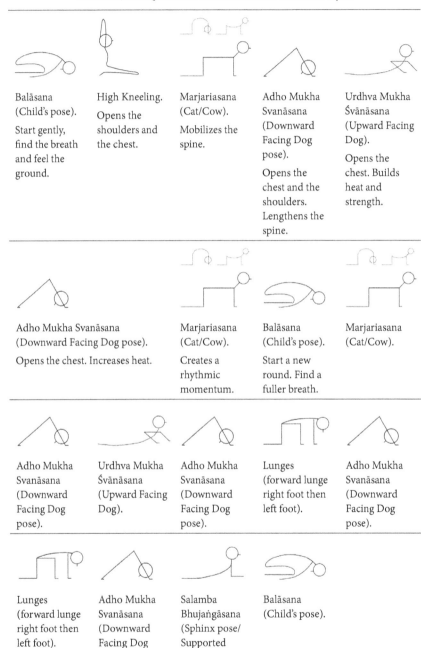

 Balāsana (Child's pose). Start gently, find the breath and feel the ground.	 High Kneeling. Opens the shoulders and the chest.	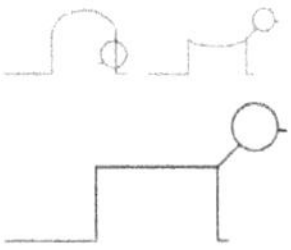 Marjariasana (Cat/Cow). Mobilizes the spine.	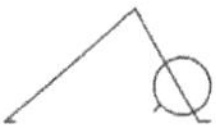 Adho Mukha Svanāsana (Downward Facing Dog pose). Opens the chest and the shoulders. Lengthens the spine.	 Urdhva Mukha Śvānāsana (Upward Facing Dog). Opens the chest. Builds heat and strength.
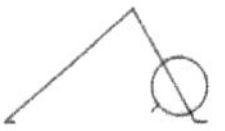 Adho Mukha Svanāsana (Downward Facing Dog pose). Opens the chest. Increases heat.		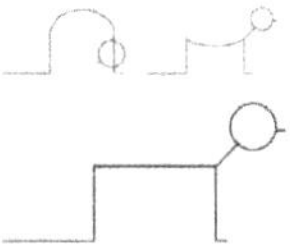 Marjariasana (Cat/Cow). Creates a rhythmic momentum.	 Balāsana (Child's pose). Start a new round. Find a fuller breath.	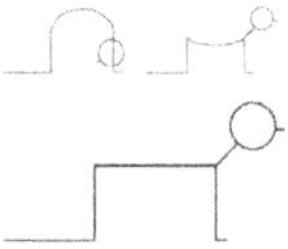 Marjariasana (Cat/Cow).
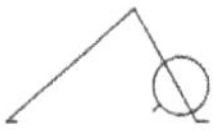 Adho Mukha Svanāsana (Downward Facing Dog pose).	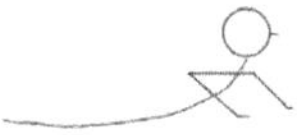 Urdhva Mukha Śvānāsana (Upward Facing Dog).	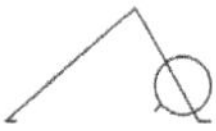 Adho Mukha Svanāsana (Downward Facing Dog pose).	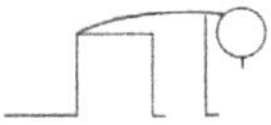 Lunges (forward lunge right foot then left foot).	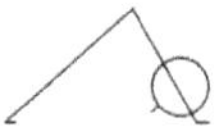 Adho Mukha Svanāsana (Downward Facing Dog pose).
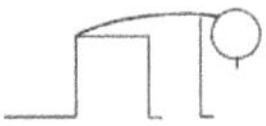 Lunges (forward lunge right foot then left foot).	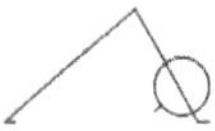 Adho Mukha Svanāsana (Downward Facing Dog pose).	 Salamba Bhujaṅgāsana (Sphinx pose/ Supported Cobra pose).	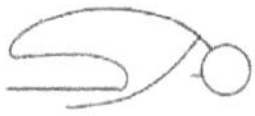 Balāsana (Child's pose).	

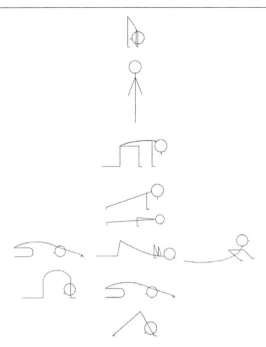

Momentum gradually increases until you are in full Sūrya Namaskara (Sun Salutation). This is a classical variation but there are other traditions and variations too. It doesn't matter which you do as long as the principles of building, heat, stamina and momentum are adhered to.

Standing poses 1–12 below can be practised in two ways: dynamically and rhythmically, holding each posture for just one or two breaths and then repeating two or three cycles, or a little more steadily, holding each posture for six to eight breaths and doing just one or two cycles.

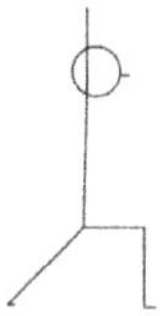

1. Warrior 1.

Emphasis on the lift and lightness without losing the strength and stability of the legs. More focus on the inhalation. Inhale on six, and exhale on four.

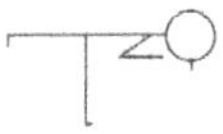

2. Vīrabhadrāsana 3 (Warrior 3).

Counterpose without losing strength.

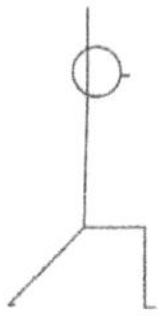

3. Vīrabhadrāsana 1 (Warrior 1).

Full and steady breathing.

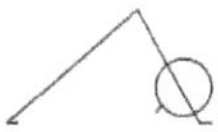

4. Adho Mukha Svanāsana (Downward Facing Dog pose).

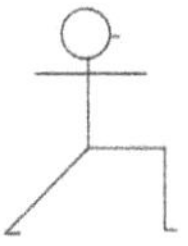

5. Vīrabhadrāsana 2 (Warrior 2).

Equal lift between front and back to create a fullness and lightness both in the chest and in the upper back.

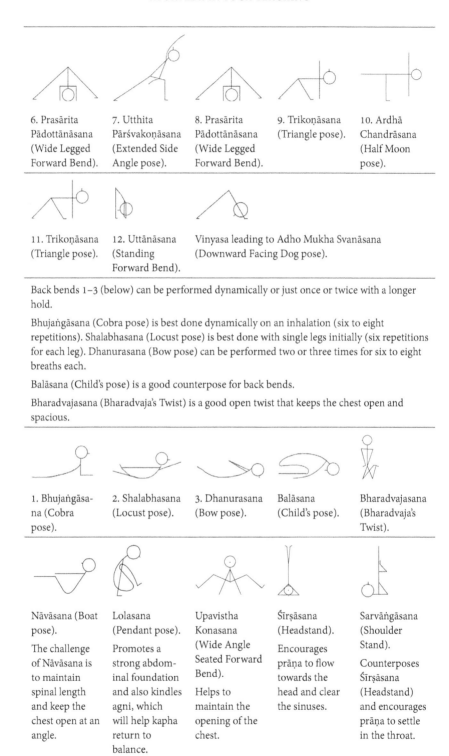

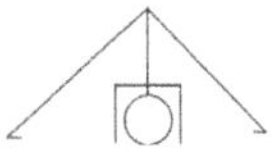

6. Prasārita Pādottānāsana (Wide Legged Forward Bend).

7. Utthita Pārśvakoṇāsana (Extended Side Angle pose).

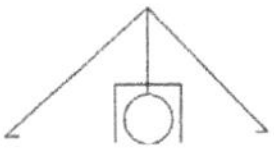

8. Prasārita Pādottānāsana (Wide Legged Forward Bend).

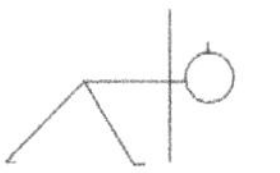

9. Trikoṇāsana (Triangle pose).

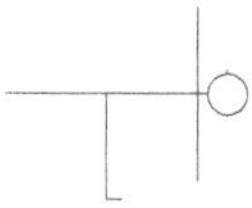

10. Ardhā Chandrāsana (Half Moon pose).

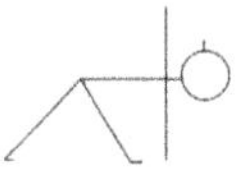

11. Trikoṇāsana (Triangle pose).

12. Uttānāsana (Standing Forward Bend).

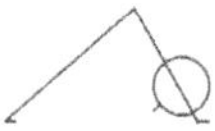

Vinyasa leading to Adho Mukha Svanāsana (Downward Facing Dog pose).

Back bends 1–3 (below) can be performed dynamically or just once or twice with a longer hold.

Bhujaṅgāsana (Cobra pose) is best done dynamically on an inhalation (six to eight repetitions). Shalabhasana (Locust pose) is best done with single legs initially (six repetitions for each leg). Dhanurasana (Bow pose) can be performed two or three times for six to eight breaths each.

Balāsana (Child's pose) is a good counterpose for back bends.

Bharadvajasana (Bharadvaja's Twist) is a good open twist that keeps the chest open and spacious.

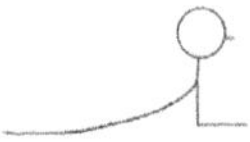

1. Bhujaṅgāsana (Cobra pose).

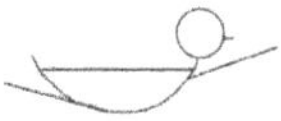

2. Shalabhasana (Locust pose).

3. Dhanurasana (Bow pose).

Balāsana (Child's pose).

Bharadvajasana (Bharadvaja's Twist).

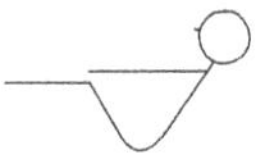

Nāvāsana (Boat pose).

The challenge of Nāvāsana is to maintain spinal length and keep the chest open at an angle.

Lolasana (Pendant pose).

Promotes a strong abdominal foundation and also kindles agni, which will help kapha return to balance.

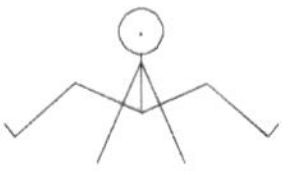

Upavistha Konasana (Wide Angle Seated Forward Bend).

Helps to maintain the opening of the chest.

Śīrṣāsana (Headstand).

Encourages prāṇa to flow towards the head and clear the sinuses.

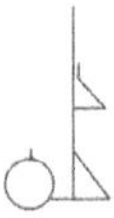

Sarvāṅgāsana (Shoulder Stand).

Counterposes Śīrṣāsana (Headstand) and encourages prāṇa to settle in the throat.

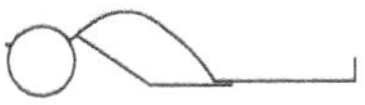	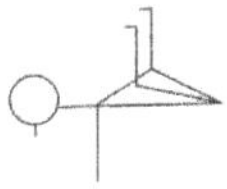	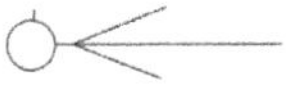
Matsyasana (Fish pose). Counterposes Sarvāṅgāsana (Shoulder Stand) and re-establishes open sensation in the chest.	Jaṭhara Parivritti (Revolved Abdomen pose). Helps realign the spine in preparation for Savasana (Corpse pose).	Savasana (Corpse pose). Whole-body integration.

—Appendix 5—

HOW TO PRACTISE JALA NETI (NASAL DOUCHING)

Precautions and disclaimer

This information is for guidance only. It is best to seek professional guidance on how to do Jala Neti if you have any medical conditions such as hypertension. Do not practise during pregnancy.

Instructions

Use a neti pot. The longer-nozzled pots are better because they make it easier to get a strong stream of water. The clean or filtered water should be at body temperature and mixed with salt: approximately one flat teaspoon per half litre of water. The salt ensures that the osmotic pressure is equal to that of the body fluids, thereby minimizing any irritation to the mucous membranes. A painful sensation suggests that there is either too little or not enough salt in the water. If you live in an area where the water is very hard, you might prefer to use soft water that is sold for use with irons.

1. Fill the neti pot with the prepared salt water.
2. Stand squarely with the legs apart, with the body weight evenly distributed between the feet, and lean forward.
3. Close the eyes for a minute or so and relax the whole body.

4. Tilt the head to one side, and back slightly.
5. Begin to breathe through the mouth.
6. Gently insert the nozzle into the nostril. There should be no force involved. The nozzle should press firmly against the side of the nostril so that no water leakage occurs.
7. Tilt the nozzle in such a way that the water runs into the nostril and not down the face. Pour half the water out of the neti pot and then change to the other nostril.
8. When the water is finished, do a few reps of Kapālabhātī *gently* to clear the nose (doing it too forcefully can push water into the sinuses or the ears).
9. Dry the nostrils thoroughly. Some residual water will remain in the sinuses for a while after the practice, so have a tissue to hand.
10. Practise Adho Mukha Svanāsana (Downward Facing Dog pose) afterwards to clear out any residual water.

—Appendix 6—

CHĀKRAS

Chākra	No of petals	Colour	Physical location	Kshetram (replace with front side)	Musical notes	Element Vayu	Yantra	Bīja mantra	Animal	Sense/ motor organ	Planet
Mūlādhāra Root	4	Deep red	Perineum Between the anus and genitals Base of the spine	Perineum Cervix	Sa	Earth Apāna	Yellow square	Laṃ	Elephant	Smell Anus	Saturn (Survival)
Svādishthāna Dwelling place of the Self	6	Orange/red	Coccyx (tail bone) Hypogastric plexus	Pubic bone	Re	Water Apāna	Silver or white crescent moon	Vaṃ	Alligator	Taste Tongue Genitals Kidneys Bladder	Jupiter (Expansion)
Manipūra City of jewels	10	Yellow	Spine behind the navel	Navel	Ga	Fire	Red inverted triangle	Raṃ	Ram	Sight Feet and legs	Mars (Power)
Anāhata Unstruck	12	Blue	Spine behind the heart	Centre of the chest	Ma	Air	Smoky six-pointed star	Yaṃ	Antelope	Touch Hands	Venus (Love)
Vishuddhi Pure	16	Purple (Blue)	Behind the throat	Pit of the throat	Pa	Space	White circle	Ham	Swan White elephant	Hearing Vocal cords	Mercury (Communi-cation)
Ājñā Master	2	Clear/grey/ indigo	Centre of the head	Eyebrow centre	Dha	Mind	Clear or grey circle	Om	Eagle	Mind	Moon (Mind)
Bindu			Back of the head, near the top		Ni		Crescent moon				
Sahasrāra Thousand petalled	1000+	Multicoloured	Crown of the head	Crown of the head	Sa		Beyond	Om			

REFERENCES

Print

Bhishagratna, K, K. (1996). *Suśruta-saṃhitā*. Varanasi: Chowkhamba Sanskrit Series Office.

Birch, J. (2018). Pre-modern Yoga Traditions and Āyurveda: Preliminary remarks on Shared Terminology, Theory and Praxis. School of Oriental and African Studies. London University. Accessed on 1/3/21 at http://hssa-journal.org.

Davies, S. (2010). *Butterflies are Free to Fly*. USA: L&G Productions LLC.

Feuerstein, G. (1990). *Encyclopaedic Dictionary of Yoga*. London: Unwin Health.

Frawley, D. (1998). *Āyurveda and the Mind*. Delhi: Motilal Banarsidass.

Frawley, D. (1999). *Yoga and Āyurveda*. Twin Lakes, WI: Lotus Press.

Frawley, D. (2000). *Ayurvedic Healing*. (Second edition.) Twin Lakes, WI: Lotus Press.

Frawley, D., Ranade, S. & Lele, A. (2003). *Āyurveda and Marma Therapy*. Twin Lakes, WI: Lotus Press.

Gregor, M. (2020). *Flashback Friday: How Many Bowel Movements Should You Have & Should You Sit, Lean, or Squat?* Accessed on 24/2/2021 at https://nutritionfacts.org/video/flashback-friday-how-many-bowel-movements-should-you-have-should-you-sit-lean-or-squat. Nutrition Facts. www.nutritionfacts.org

Jarmey, C., Bouratinos, I. (2008). *A Practical Guide to Acu-points*. Chichester: Lotus Publishing.

Lad, V. (2002). *Textbook of Āyurveda*, Volume 1. Albuquerque, NM: The Ayurvedic Press. (p.86)

Lad, V. & Durve, A. (2008). *Marma Points of Āyurveda*. Albuquerque, NM: The Ayurvedic Press.

Lipton, B. (2015). *Is there a way to change subconscious patterns?* Accessed on 31/3/2021 at www.brucelipton.com/there-way-change-subconscious-patterns.

Mitra, J. (1998). *Suśruta-saṃhitā: Sūtrasthāna*. Chapter XXV. Varanasi: Chowkhamba Sanskrit Series Office.

Muktibodhananda, Swami (1998). *Haṭha Yoga Pradīpikā*. (Third edition.) Bihar: Yoga Publications Trust.

Murthy, S. (1999). *Vaghbata's Aṣṭāṅga Hṛdaya*. Sūtrasthāna. Varanasi: Krishnadas Academy.

National Centre for Biotechnology Information (2009). *Saline Nasal Irrigation for Upper Respiratory Conditions*. Accessed on 24/2/2021 at www.ncbi.nlm.nih.gov/pmc/articles/PMC2778074/.

News Medical (2018). *pH in the Human Body*. Accessed on 18/2/2021 at www.news-medical.net/health/pH-in-the-Human-Body.aspx.

O'Neill, S. (2017). *Yoga Teaching Handbook*. London: Jessica Kingsley Publishers.

O'Neill, S. (2019). *Yoga Student Handbook*. London: Jessica Kingsley Publishers.

Satyananda Saraswati, Swami (1973). *Sūrya Namaskar*. Bihar: Bihar School of Yoga.

Satyananda Saraswati, Swami. (1976) *Yoga Nidrā*. (Fifth edition.) Bihar: Bihar School of Yoga.

Satyananda Saraswati, Swami (1997) *Āsana, Prāṇāyāma, Mudrā, Bandha*. Bihar: Bihar School of Yoga.

Satyananda Saraswati, Swami (2004). *Nine Principal Upaniṣads*. Bihar: Yoga Publications Trust.

Sharma, P.V. (2000). *Caraka-saṃhitā*. (Sixth edition.) Varanasi: Chaukhambha Orientalia.

Sivananda, Swami (1991). *Kundalini Yoga*. (Ninth edition.) Tehri-Garhwal: Divine Life Society.

Three Initiates. (2018). *The Kybalion, Hermetic Philosophy*. UK: Perennial Press.

Wisdom Library (2020). *Kapha*. Accessed on 18/2/2021 at www.wisdomlib.org/definition/ka.

Wisdom Library (2021). *Pitta*. Accessed on 18/2/2021 at www.wisdomlib.org/definition/pitta.

Wisdom Library (2021) *Prasada*. Accessed on 18/2/2021 https://www.wisdomlib.org/definition/prasada.

Wisdom Library (2021). *Snigdha, Snigdhā*. Accessed on 18/2/2021 at www.wisdomlib.org/definition/snigdha.

Wisdom Library (2021). *Tarpaka*. Accessed on 18/2/2021 at www.wisdomlib.org/definition/tarpaka.

Wisdom Library (n.d.) *Kṛkāṭikāaṭika*. Accessed on 2/9/2020 at www.wisdomlib.org/definition/KṛkāṭikāKaṭika.

Wisdom Library (n.d.) *Māṇibandha*. Accessed on 2/9/2020 at www.wisdomlib.org/definition/Māṇibandha.

Wisdom Library (n.d.) *Vishnu*. Accessed on 2/9/2020 at www.wisdomlib.org/definition/LohitākṣaLohitākṣa.

Yogapedia (2018). *Sanātana Dharma*. Accessed on 18/2/2021 at www.yogapedia.com/definition/6240/Sanātana-dharma.

Further reading

Frawley, D. and Summerfield Kozak, S. (2001). *Yoga for your Type*. Twin Lakes, WI: Lotus Press.

Lad, V. (1984). *Āyurveda: The Science of Self-Healing*. Delhi: Motilal Banarsidass.

O'Neill, S. (2017). *Yoga Teaching Handbook*. London: Jessica Kingsley Publishers.

Satyananda Saraswati, Swami (1997). *Āsana, Prāṇāyāma Mudrā, Bandha*. Bihar: Bihar School of Yoga.

Svoboda, R. (1992). *Āyurveda: Life, Health and Longevity*. Albuquerque, NM: The Ayurvedic Press.

INDEX